THE PSYCHIATRIC DILEMMA
OF ADOLESCENCE

THE

PSYCHIATRIC

DILEMMA OF

ADOLESCENCE

JAMES F. MASTERSON, Jr.
M. D.

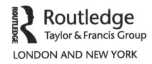

Routledge
Taylor & Francis Group

LONDON AND NEW YORK

To THOSE WHO HAVE TROD THIS PATH BEFORE, AND TO MY
LEGACY TO THE FUTURE, J. F., RICHARD, AND NANCY

SECOND PRINTING

First published by BRUNNER/MAZEL, INC.

Published 2014 by Routledge
2 Park Square, Milton Park, Abingdon, Oxfordshire OX14 4RN
711 Third Avenue, New York, NY 10017

First issued in paperback 2014

Routledge is an imprint of the Taylor and Francis Group, an informa business

Library of Congress Cataloging in Publication Data

Masterson, James F.
  The psychiatric dilemma of adolescence.

  Reprint. Originally published: Boston : Little,
Brown, 1967.
  Bibliography: p.
  Includes index.
  1. Adolescent psychopathology — Diagnosis —
Longitudinal studies. 2. Adolescent psychopathology —
Longitudinal studies. 3. Adolescent psychology —
Longitudinal studies. I. Title.
RJ503.M3 1984   616.89'0088055   83-24039
ISBN 0-87630-356-4

ISBN 13: 978-0-87630-356-6 (hbk)
ISBN 13: 978-1-138-00441-2 (pbk)

INTRODUCTION TO 1984 EDITION

THIS VOLUME, FIRST PUBLISHED in 1967 and reissued now in 1984, is addressed to students of adolescent psychopathology in general and to sudents of the borderline and narcissistic personality disorders in particular. It was the first systematic research to challenge and place in perspective the then prevalent "adolescent turmoil" theory: the growth process of adolescence was producing symptoms which would subside as the patient grew older. This view had led to a tendency to deny the seriousness of psychopathology and, therefore, to postpone necessary treatment.

The findings, of course, were almost the opposite: Most of the adolescents (particularly those with schizophrenia or a personality disorder) did not "grow out of it" but got worse as they grew older.

Every study of this subject since 1967 has replicated these findings. They remain as valid today as when first published. It is as important now as it was then that the therapist use this understanding in his clinical evaluations.

The book presents extensive clinical cases, free of any theoretical bias, which are followed up five years later. This overview of a wide spectrum of adolescent psychopathology allows the reader to make his own evaluations and test them against the follow-up results, thereby honing his observational and diagnostic skills.

Beyond that, the findings presented here led me into a 28-year path of investigation of the so-called personality disorders, which resulted in the emergence of a developmental, object-relations approach to the borderline and personality disorders which dramatically improved therapeutic techniques and clinical results. This volume then represents the starting point of the evolution of that concept. It was the first of what eventually became a trilogy of books on what I called "the borderline adolescent."

This book introduced the problem: The adolescent with a personality disorder didn't grow out of it. It even provided hints of our future understanding by showing that depression in adolescents with a personality disorder increases rather than decreases as they get older (see p. 111). It also showed that the key prognostic determinant was not the symptoms but the underlying pathologic character traits.

The second book, *Treatment of the Borderline Adolescent* (John Wiley & Sons, 1972), described a study that developed treatment techniques for these character traits using a developmental, object-relations theory. The third book, *From Borderline Adolescent to Functioning Adult: The Test of Time* (Brunner/Mazel, 1981), reported a follow-up study of the patients treated in 1972. This evaluates the effectiveness of the therapeutic approach. This same approach was then also applied to the borderline and narcissistic personality disorder in the adult. Consequently, this volume represents the fountainhead and starting point of the entire work. Since the best way to understand an idea is to trace its evolution, those interested in the present-day volumes on the borderline and narcissistic personality disorders will find this volume of interest.

J.F.M.
January, 1984

PREFACE

THE PSYCHIATRIC DILEMMA of adolescence is created by the clinical difficulty in determining whether a symptomatic adolescent suffers from a psychiatric illness and requires treatment or from so-called adolescent turmoil that will subside with further growth. This dilemma is further enhanced by current psychoanalytic theory, which stresses that adolescent turmoil not only causes psychiatric symptoms to be common and temporary in most adolescents, but also causes psychiatric syndromes to be ill-defined, difficult to diagnose, and transient; the patients often "grow out of their difficulties" later in life.

This book, written for the clinician who treats adolescents, provides some answers to this dilemma by reporting the major part of a longitudinal study of adolescent patients and controls which investigated the relationship of this theory to clinical reality. The book deals with such questions as: What are the relationships of "adolescent turmoil" to psychiatric illness? What are the diagnostic difficulties in adolescent patients? Can they be defined and categorized? Are they resolved, or do they continue over the course of time? What happens to these patients as they proceed through the years of their adolescence? Do they show wide fluctuations in their symptomatology? Are they truly "just in a phase," and do they, as theory suggests, grow out of their difficulties? And, finally, how do psychiatrically ill adolescents compare with those who are healthy?

Many of the findings ran counter to theory. For example, the initial diagnostic difficulties lay not in the choice between an adjustment reaction of adolescence and a psychiatric illness, but rather in determining the exact clinical diagnosis of the illness. Far from growing out of their difficulties, the majority of the patients continued to suffer from symptoms and to be markedly impaired in functioning. The minority who functioned well did so by finding better ways of handling their conflicts. However, the persistence of these conflicts together with the development of pathological character traits suggests that they remain quite vulnerable to future stress. In addition, the patients differed substantially from their healthy counterparts. In a concluding synthesis, the book reexamines the relationship of adolescent turmoil to psychiatric illness, qualifies current theory in the light of the findings, and

vii

offers some guiding concepts for future confrontations with this clinical problem.

I would like to emphasize that the findings presented, many of which are contradictory to the current psychoanalytic theory of adolescent turmoil, came as quite a surprise, since my own orientation, though eclectic, is predominantly psychoanalytic.

The research for this book was supported by the Health Research Council of New York City, the Cornell Program in Social Psychiatry, and the Foundations Fund for Research in Psychiatry. I hope this book will temper the misgivings of many granting agencies, notoriously loathe to underwrite such work, and that it will encourage them to support actively a type of endeavor that is essential to the progress of psychiatry.

J. F. M.

ACKNOWLEDGMENTS

I OWE SO MUCH to so many that it is difficult to know where to begin. The research staff listed below, who bore the burden of the work, labored long and well in a true scientific spirit. Although all of them at one time or another participated in every phase of the study, Dr. Kenneth Tucker and Mrs. Gloria Berk were particularly involved in the organizational phase and Drs. Murray Kofkin and Harry Wallenstein and Miss Eileen Corrigan in the control phase. Misses Antonia Washburne and Eileen Corrigan in addition greatly lessened my burdens by assisting in the administration of the project.

A number of consultants contributed to the project. Dr. Alexander Leighton, serving as an occasional consultant, was always a source of support and at one point furnished funds to tide the control study over a difficult period. Dr. Dorothea Leighton helped to plan and organize the study. Dr. Oskar Diethelm, head of the department of Psychiatry, Cornell University Medical College, during most of the study, provided essential administrative support and also helped to secure funds. Dr. John Harding, the principal statistical consultant, showed enormous patience and diligence in instructing the author in the complexities of statistics. As the study moved into the final clinical phase, Drs. Daniel Offer, Willard Hendrickson, and Philip Escoll gave me the benefit of their clinical experience by reviewing some of the findings. Drs. Offer and Hendrickson also reviewed the first draft of the manuscript and made many helpful comments. In addition, Dr. William Lulow read the manuscript.

The analysis on which the findings in this book are based and the writing itself are the responsibility of the author. Whatever readability and style the work contains is in no small measure due to two consultants, both of Cornell University Medical College: Milton Zisowitz, Lecturer in Medical Writing, who taught me to value precise writing and edited every chapter, and Miss Helen Goodell, Research Associate, Department of Neurology, who also edited every chapter and who served as an efficient sounding board. It is not possible to acknowledge individually the many secretaries who participated in this project over the years. I would like therefore to thank them all in the person of the last, Mrs. Nancy Scanlan, whose help was invaluable as much for her dedication and enthusiasm as for her sterling secretarial ability. Finally, I am grateful to S. A., without whose help the book would probably have remained a figment of my imagination.

*Research Staff: The Symptomatic Adolescent Research Project**

Project Director
    James F. Masterson, Jr., M.D.
    Associate Professor of Clinical Psychiatry
    Cornell University Medical College

Psychiatrists
    Kenneth Tucker, M.D.
    Instructor in Psychiatry
    Cornell University Medical College

    Murray Kofkin, M.D.
    Instructor in Psychiatry
    Cornell University Medical College

    Harry Wallenstein, M.D.
    Instructor in Psychiatry
    Cornell University Medical College

Social Workers
    Gloria Berk, B.A., M.S.S.
    Psychiatric Social Worker
    Payne Whitney Psychiatric Clinic

    Eileen Corrigan, B.A., M.S.S.
    Psychiatric Social Worker
    Payne Whitney Psychiatric Clinic

    Antonia Washburne, B.A., M.S.S.
    Psychiatric Social Worker
    Payne Whitney Psychiatric Clinic

* All appointments are those held at the time of the study.

Statistical Assistants
   Cho Shirae, B.S.
   Nancy Payne, B.S.
   Martin Goldman, B.S.

Consultants
 Clinical
   Willard Hendrickson, M.D.
   Associate Professor of Adolescent Psychiatry
   University of Michigan

   Daniel Offer, M.D.
   Associate Director
   Institute for Psychosomatic and Psychiatric Research and Training
   Michael Reese Medical Center, Chicago

   Philip Escoll, M.D.
   Assistant Professor of Clinical Psychiatry
   University of Pennsylvania

 Methodology
   Alexander H. Leighton, M.D.
   Professor of Psychiatry (Social Psychiatry)
   Cornell University Medical College

   Dorothea Leighton, M.D.
   Clinical Associate Professor of Psychiatry (Social Psychiatry)
   Cornell University Medical College

   John Harding, Ph.D.
   Associate Professor of Child Development and Family
      Relationships
   Cornell University Medical College

CONTENTS

xiii

SECTION I

THE PROBLEM AND
THE APPROACH

CHAPTER 1

THE PROBLEM: "IT'S JUST A PHASE"

> I cannot forecast to you the action of Russia. It is a
> riddle wrapped in a mystery inside an enigma.
> —Winston S. Churchill: radio
> broadcast, October 1, 1939

THE WORDS WINSTON CHURCHILL USED to describe his reaction to Soviet Russia also aptly describe the reaction of the psychiatrist when he must evaluate the symptomatic adolescent. He is faced with an apparently insoluble riddle—that of differentiating between psychiatric illness, which requires treatment, and "adolescent turmoil," which may subside with growth, the development of maturity, and the passage of time. To illustrate the difficulties involved in this task, and therefore the clinical dilemma that prompted this research, let us retrace with you the voyage which we began in December, 1956, and end on these pages. Let the port of embarkation be the office of the psychiatrist faced with the symptomatic adolescent: the first port of call is a visit with our colleagues; the second is a review of the American Psychiatric Association's *Diagnostic and Statistical Manual of Mental Disorders*; the third is a review of the literature; and the final destination is the findings published here.

Imagine yourself as the psychiatrist—before you an obese seventeen-year-old girl, a high school junior. With persistent and skillful questioning you get the following history from this troubled young girl, who has been referred to the clinic because of her increasing difficulties in school. Six months prior to the interview after a discussion about boys with her girl friends, she reluctantly tells you, she first became aware of anxiety and guilt about sexual feelings. Several months later she did poorly on college board examinations. Her previously mild anxiety, guilt, and depression became worse, as did her sense of inadequacy and of inability to concentrate. She became increasingly anxious in social situations, to such a degree that she began to withdraw from social contacts, feeling that no one could like her. She confesses to a great desire to have her father like her, but can only bitterly resent him because he shows no concern for or interest in her. She

3

clings to an overindulgent mother and overprotective sister, neither of whom has an intelligent sympathy for the patient's dark moods and persistent obesity. There is a past history, throughout the first eight grades of school, of obesity and a conduct disorder manifested by rebelliousness against her teachers though she managed to pass her academic work. Although at age thirteen the conduct disorder subsided, the obesity continued.

On this first examination she is preoccupied with guilt feelings about sex and her resentment toward her father. She appears immature, anxious, and depressed, and possibly has a blunted affect. Tears are close to the surface. Expression of her feelings is perfunctory and communication guarded, but there is no evidence of a thinking disorder.

As we tried to put this clinical picture together in order to make some practical and necessary decisions, a number of questions came to our minds. First, although she had had symptoms for some time, there had been a recent upsurge related to sexual preoccupations. Could this and perhaps the depression and conflict with the father be related to adolescent turmoil—were they likely, therefore, to subside with the passage of time and the development of her individuality and independence? Or did she have a psychiatric illness which required treatment? If the latter, what was the diagnosis—schizophrenia, personality disorder, or psychoneurosis? No doubt adolescent turmoil, if it can simulate a psychiatric illness, can also color or intensify the clinical picture of one. Which of this patient's symptoms had serious prognostic import and which did not? What would her clinical picture look like after adolescence? How common were these symptoms in adolescents who never see a psychiatrist? Was the conflict with the father related to the need for emancipation, or was it a more serious, lifelong conflict, one in which she had chronically felt deprived of love? At this point in our ruminations we wondered how we could make a rational decision without answers to some of these questions, which actually all boil down to a single theme: the effect of adolescent turmoil on the clinical manifestations and outcome of those with a psychiatric illness, as well as its effect on normal adolescents.

When we stopped at the first port of call by repairing to our colleagues for help, we found that not only did they share our confusion but some of them had tried to resolve it by using, in many cases inappropriately, the APA manual's diagnostic category "adjustment re-action of adolescence" [2]. As a result many hospitals, our own in-cluded, are filled with adolescents with such differing disorders as schizophrenia and personality disorder, all carrying the same label: "adjustment reaction of adolescence." We began to feel that this diagnostic category, defined for transient reactions related to growth, had become a refuge and a "wastebasket" which prevented a real comprehension of the underlying issues. We then decided to examine more thoroughly this wastebasket category—devised, no doubt, in an effort to handle the very dilemma we have presented.

The APA manual lists three criteria of "adjustment reaction of adolescence": First, the clinical picture is that of a psychiatric illness which can take any form; second, the symptoms must be related to the growth process of adolescence; and third, the symptoms should be transient. Immediately some objections come to mind. For example, how can one tell whether symptoms are going to be transient or not when the patient is in the midst of a psychiatric syndrome? Certainly since there is great doubt about the nature of the growth process of adolescence, it is also often difficult to decide whether symptoms may be related to it.

Having left the port of embarkation and made one stop, we are now both metaphorically and realistically at sea. Perhaps our next stop, a review of the literature, will enable us to check our compass and get a more secure sense of direction. This port of call is explored for some specific reasons. We should like to know what adolescent disorders have been described and later followed up, and what clinical pictures fitted the characterization of "just in a phase."

Here we find a problem unique to the field of psychiatry. Until recently the clinical psychiatrist has shown very little interest in study-ing the processes of growth and development in adolescence. Conse-quently his reports consist primarily of descriptions of clinical illnesses in hospitalized patients, touching lightly if at all on the question of adolescent turmoil but more often including a follow-up. The strength of these reports lies in their fairly large numbers, the presence of follow-up, and the focus on clinical descriptions. Their weakness lies in the inadequate consideration given to the dynamic aspects of adolescent turmoil and in the concentration on hospitalized patients.

The domain of growth and development, on the other hand, and therefore of adolescent turmoil, has appeared to be mainly that of the psychoanalyst. The strength of the analytic reports lies in their detailed theoretical consideration of the processes underlying growth and development, including adolescent turmoil and its relationship to psychopathology. Their weakness lies first in the fact that *adolescence* is often used as a generic term without being adequately differentiated for various diagnostic categories. Second, although clinical illustrations are presented, they are few in number, and discussion is focused on dynamics and defense mechanisms with less emphasis on clinical description. And finally, there is rarely an adequate follow-up.

So we have an apparently unbridgeable chasm. On the one shore are the reports of clinical psychiatrists on hospitalized patients, presenting rather large numbers of clinical descriptions and follow-ups, but with inadequate consideration of adolescent turmoil. On the other shore are the reports of psychoanalysts, with wholly adequate consideration of the dynamics and defense mechanisms of adolescent turmoil, but covering small numbers of patients and lacking follow-up.

Let us turn to the psychiatric reports first. In 1957, as part of a follow-up study of hospitalized adolescents, we reviewed the literature describing psychiatric illness in adolescence and its outcome [45, 46]. Since psychiatric research was applied late to the study of adolescence, few reports were available at that time. To summarize the conclusions we derived from these previous studies, it was found that adolescents with schizophrenia and organic reactions have a poor outcome, while those with affective disorders or psychoneurosis have a good outcome. The most cogent reference to adolescent turmoil suggested that it may precipitate an acute confusional psychosis in schizophrenic adolescents who later have a good outcome. Since 1957 the increased interest in this long-neglected area has resulted in a flood of clinical reports, usually dealing with treatment [6, 11, 32, 35, 37, 42, 53, 55, 65, 81], psychodynamics, and pathology [3, 4, 5, 23, 36, 40, 52, 56, 68–70, 75–77, 80, 83]. Other recent follow-up psychiatric studies of larger groups including adolescents are those by O'Neal and Robins [61–63, 66–67] and the Gluecks' classic study of delinquency and criminality [30] and some follow-up studies have been made of adolescents per se [10, 18, 78–79, 82]. Though these studies are helpful in further delineating the characteristics of psychiatric illness in adolescence, they were not designed to give an appropriate answer to the questions we have raised.

Crossing the chasm to the psychoanalytic literature we find that, like clinical psychiatry, psychoanalysis also has come relatively recently to the study of adolescence. It began with Freud's three essays on sexuality [28] followed by Ernest Jones' article on "Some Problems of Adolescence" [38] and then the work of Aichhorn [1], Bernfeld [12–15], and Anna Freud [24, 25]. In the postwar years, particularly in the United States, the published research on adolescence has mushroomed. Since this is not a psychoanalytic treatise, we refer the reader to two excellent reviews of the psychoanalytic literature on adolescence by Spiegel in 1951 [73] and by Anna Freud in 1958 [26]. It suffices for our purpose to say that we found a rather striking agreement as to a psychoanalytic theory for this clinical dilemma, by such authors as Erickson [22], Eissler [21], Josselyn [39], Blos [16], Anna Freud [26], and Helene Deutsch [19]. We shall summarize the theory, including some quotations from the authors to dramatize the weight of psychoanalytic opinion on this issue.

The ego structure in adolescence is in a state of marked flux and weakness owing to the growth process. This condition of flux causes (1) psychiatric syndromes, when present, to be vague and ill defined and (2) to be unstable, with patients shifting from one category of disorder to another. (3) Often only follow-up of later developments in the patient's life can determine whether a given symptom picture represented psychopathology or was merely an intensification of the difficulties of adolescence. A final facet of the theory suggests that (4) psychiatric symptoms are common and transient in most adolescents.

For example, Anna Freud [26] writes, "adolescence is by its nature an interruption of peaceful growth and the upholding of a steady equilibrium during this process is in itself abnormal. . . . The adolescent manifestations of growth come close to the symptom formations of the neurotic, psychotic or dissocial order and merge almost imperceptibly into borderline states, initial, frustrated or fully fledged forms of almost all the illnesses. Consequently, the differential diagnosis between these adolescent upsets and true pathology becomes a difficult task."

Erickson [22] suggests that, "we look at adolescence not as an affliction but as a normative process, a normal phase of increased conflict characterized by seeming fluctuation in the ego strength and also by a high growth potential. What under prejudiced scrutiny may appear to be the onset of a neurosis often is but an aggravated crisis which might prove to be self-liquidating and in fact contributive to the process of identity formation."

Peter Blos [16] in his book on adolescence writes that "prediction studies would help us to understand and evaluate the non-pathological aspects of this stage in development during which the personality normally shows many apparently pathognomic features."

Helene Deutsch [19] in her *Psychology of Women* summarizes her opinion: "Only subsequent developments can show whether pathological phenomena are involved in such cases or merely intensified difficulties of adolescence."

The diagnostic difficulty is further referred to by Irene Josselyn [39]: "Before diagnosis is offered, the total picture, both in detail and in time, should be known. A typical adolescent may present a picture of hysteria while the history indicates that a month ago his behavior was typically impulsive. Next month he may appear as a compulsive-neurotic. In addition, islands of psychotic-like behavior are not unusual during adolescence."

Eissler [21] also refers to this problem when he says that "adolescent psychopathology switches from one form to another, sometimes in the course of weeks or months, but also from day to day. The symptoms manifested by such patients may be neurotic at one time and almost psychotic at another, and sudden acts of delinquency may occur only to be followed by a phase of perverted sexual activity."

On this third port of call before the longest lap of the voyage, we found some information which helped us to set the compass. We found unanimous agreement among psychoanalytic theorists about this clinical dilemma. Nevertheless, we were left with some rather gnawing doubts. In these articles the authors slip readily from talking about adolescence generically—and therefore, we assume, about normal growth and development—to a specific type of clinical problem, discussing it in terms of defenses and dynamics with less emphasis on clinical description. Are we to assume, then, that these theories, probably for the most part derived from the study of psychoneurotics, can be applied equally well to patients in other diagnostic categories? Or are we victims of the chasm in the literature between the two disciplines? For example, does adolescent turmoil cause diagnostic difficulty in adolescents who are schizophrenic or in those with a personality disorder? Does it merely intensify these conditions, leaving hope that the patients may later grow out of their difficulty? Just who are the patients whose adolescent turmoil is "a phase"? We will attempt to bridge the chasm, to reconcile the conflicting theories, and to find a synthesis that can be applied to the patients seen most commonly by clinical psychiatrists.

Now we can leave our last port of call with a firm compass setting. We have decided to ask some concrete questions amenable to research: What are the diagnostic difficulties in adolescent outpatients? Can they be recognized, defined, and categorized? How are they resolved, or do they continue over the course of time? What are the relationships of adolescent turmoil to psychiatric illness? What happens to these patients through the years of their adolescence? Do they show wide fluctuations in their symptomatology? Are they truly "just in a phase," and do they, as theory suggests, grow out of their difficulties? What is the fate of such specific symptoms as depression and acting-out? Is family conflict related to adolescent turmoil or to more persistent underlying problems? How do psychiatrically ill adolescents compare with those who are healthy?

In the next chapter we specify more concretely the compass setting by describing our method of approach. Then in the remaining chapters we bring the reader to his final destination, the setting forth of our findings, a reexamination of the relationship of adolescent turmoil to psychiatric illness together with some guiding concepts that may be helpful for future confrontations with this troublesome problem.

CHAPTER 2

METHOD: CLINICAL AND SYSTEMATIC

> I went to the woods because I wished to live de-
> liberately, to front only the essential facts of life,
> and see if I could not learn what it had to teach . . .
> —Thoreau: *Walden*

THE PURPOSE OF the project, which was exploratory and descriptive in character, was mainly to break ground in the complicated area of the dilemma of adolescence, to sketch out boundaries and provide clinical hypotheses for future studies of more specific design. The project was designed to be a five-year study of 101 adolescent outpatients and a similar five-year study of a matched group of 101 controls or nonpatients. This book is devoted primarily to the patient study, which began in December, 1956, and was concluded in 1962, the subsequent time being spent in analyzing and reporting. A part of the control study [49, 51], focused on the last element of the theory, began in 1961 and is still in progress. It is partially reported in Chapters 13 and 14.

To provide a background for our study, it is necessary to describe two conflicting views about psychiatric research that are a result of the marked advances in the technology of the physical sciences [44]. These advances, far outdistancing those of the behavioral sciences, have tempted the latter to borrow techniques from the former, to minimize the methodologic pitfalls in clinical research. This has created a conflict between two points of view. The one we call the clinical, stresses the stochastic nature of the material and emphasizes the importance of the observations and interpretations of the individual observer. The other, considered more scientific by its proponents, we call the systematic; it stresses the need to control bias and emphasizes the use of more than one observer, careful definitions of the variables to be studied, and the employment of coding schemes, data analysis, and statistical probability calculations.

Those favoring the latter view argue that the objectivity of clinical research is limited by the bias of the individual observer, whether based on his personality characteristics or his theoretical persuasion, and by lack of adequate definition of the variables to be studied. In addition, they assert that these defects leave conclusions subject to the idiosyncratic views of the researcher and make replication difficult. They contend that the systematic approach is more scientific because it minimizes individual bias, provides adequate definition of the variables to be studied, minimizes the idiosyncratic views of the researchers, and therefore makes replication easier.

The clinician counters with the argument that the systematic approach, though admittedly reducing individual bias, is most effective when one or two variables can be isolated and controlled, and hence is not always appropriate to clinical material, which is complex and involves many variables operating at the same time. He would further assert that the clinical approach, though having its methodologic problems, is no less scientific than the systematic and is the only method suitable to use with clinical material. Clearly, the choice between these two views depends upon the nature of the phenomena to be studied and the questions to be asked. For example, if we were going to study a thousand patients to determine the prevalence of symptomatology, the systematic method might be more appropriate, whereas if we wished to study all the determinants of a symptom complex, then the clinical would be in order.

The control study, asking questions regarding symptomatology and impairment of functioning in two different groups, argued strongly for the systematic method, while the longitudinal aspect of both studies, focusing on the comprehensive clinical picture, favored use of the clinical approach. Therefore, we decided to try both methods, hoping to test their limits. It seems wise, before going on, to report our final impressions of the two approaches. We did find the systematic approach valuable in situations in which we were comparing isolated variables in two different groups (see patients and controls, Chapters 13 and 14). In the longitudinal study, however, the isolation of variables involved in the systematic approach lessened the important contribution to meaning of the relationship of all of the variables acting one upon another at one point in time. Therefore, the findings reported in this book except for Chapters 13 and 14 are based on the clinical approach, which consisted of a case-by-case clinical review, integrating all the data into a comprehensive clinical picture of the onset, course, and outcome of the illnesses. Some of the personal bias to which this method is susceptible can be minimized by a personal analysis in which the author was engaged throughout the study. In addition, what the results may lose from unrecognized unconscious bias they may gain from the judgment and intuition of an experienced clinician applied to an evaluation of all the variables. The findings reported in Chapters 13 and 14 are based on the systematic method, the details of which are in the Appendix.

Selection of Cases

The initial study group consisted of 101 patients, ages twelve to eighteen, consecutive admissions accepted for consultation by the adolescent outpatient clinic between December 31, 1956, and February, 1958. These were approximately one-half of the 227 who applied for admission during that time. Referrals came from school, family, family doctor, court, social agencies, and the New York Hospital. It was our admission policy to see in consultation any patient of at least average intelligence who did not have a long history of previous treatment, who was not openly negativistic, whose parents were willing to participate, and who might benefit from outpatient treatment. When the family applied, the social worker first interviewed the mother, then discussed the findings with the psychiatrist, who decided whether or not to see the patient. (Table 1 gives general diagnostic impressions of the types of patients automatically excluded from our group.)

Table 1.   Patients Who Applied But Were Not Seen

Classification	No. of Patients
Retarded	11
Juvenile delinquent	24
Psychotic	19
Behavior problems without motivation	28
Psychoneurosis with extreme family conflict	18
Psychoneurotic symptoms with social difficulty	13
Learning difficulty	4
Brain damage or other serious physical impairments	5
Wrong age	2
Problems other than psychological	2
Total	126

Forty-one per cent of these had acting-out problems, 25 per cent had psychoneurotic difficulties, 15 per cent were psychotic, and 9 per cent were retarded.

The seventy-two patients (forty-seven boys and twenty-five girls) reported here represent that part of the 101 who were followed for the five-year period. The sex ratio of two boys to one girl compares with a larger group of adolescents (380) seen in the outpatient department, where the ratio was three to one. As Table 1 indicates, admission policies reduced the number in the study group with severe acting-out problems.

Initial Examination Procedures

The patients were seen by two psychiatrists, one of whom took 45 minutes to an hour for the interview, the other 30 minutes. The interview technique was similar to that used in a psychiatric consultation. The psychiatrist began with the present illness and then reviewed the patient's past history; the order of topics was not fixed, and an effort was made to obtain the desired information while preserving the flexibility necessary to pursue clinical leads as they arose. One of the two psychiatrists also interviewed the parent: mother in eighty-one cases, both parents in five cases, father in seven cases, a parent surrogate in four cases, and no parent in four cases. The interview with the parent focused on the patient's symptoms, past history, and family relationship. The parent's background and personality were only superficially investigated. Following the interview, the two doctors conferred to record disagreements in both observations and interpretations.

To promote the consistency and uniformity of clinical observation, examination forms* were filled out, usually after the interviews. The patient form contained categories for chief complaint, history of present illness, effect of symptoms on school and social functioning, past history, and attitude of patient to mother and father. The form for the parent focused on the patient's symptoms, developmental history, and relationship with the parent.

Ideally, to know whether a patient has "grown out of his difficulties," one should have followed him until the end of the adolescent

* See Appendix, under Clinical Method.

phase of his development. The average age of our patients on first examination was sixteen. Practical considerations led us to choose a follow-up interval of five years, which placed most of them chronologically past their adolescent years, even though many emotionally might not have completed the adolescent phase of development—which, in any event, may be as much a conceptual as a realistic condition. We also decided to do an interim follow-up examination after two and a half years in the hope that it might provide some information on fluctuations during adolescence. In the two-and-a-half-year examination, sixty-four patients and mothers were seen; in the remaining fourteen cases, only the mother was interviewed. Of the twenty-three not seen, six could not be located. Of the seventeen located but not seen, thirteen refused and four were not available (out of state). In the five-year examination, seventy patients and mothers were seen, and in the remaining ten cases only the mother was interviewed. Of the ten cases in which only the mother was seen, eight were excluded from this report because we felt the information was inadequate. This report, then, is based on seventy-two of the eighty. Of the twenty-one cases not seen, ten could not be located, and of the eleven located but not seen, seven refused and four were unavailable.

Since the interviews had to be scheduled at the patients' convenience, so many practical problems arose for the two psychiatrists that, after a trial series of interviews to establish that the observations of the social worker were consistent with those of both psychiatrists, we changed the method of interviewing from two psychiatrists to a psychiatrist and a social worker. The psychiatrist reviewed the previous record to prepare for the interview, but his chief responsibility was a thorough current psychiatric evaluation. The social worker's principal functions, in addition to interviewing the parent, were to insure a detailed follow-up on previous findings and to administer a comprehensive questionnaire designed to cover a broad spectrum of symptomatology, as described below.

At the conclusion of the initial interview, we became aware that the psychiatrist was more likely to pursue present florid symptomatology in depth rather than to search carefully for all other symptom patterns. For subsequent interviews, we devised a questionnaire to cover the entire spectrum of psychopathology (see Appendix). Therefore, the two follow-up interviews differed from the initial one in the use of a questionnaire which helped us to focus as much on obtaining all symptom patterns as on presenting symptomatology. It brought to light, we felt, a greater number of certain symptom patterns, such as obsessive-compulsive, psychophysiologic, and hypochondriacal. However, although these were found to be more common on the follow-up than on the initial interview, we had less confidence in the increase, for if a questionnaire had been used on the initial interview these same symptom patterns would probably also have been shown to be more common on that interview. Though we cannot put much stock in the increase in symptom patterns, we can no doubt have more confidence in their disappearance on follow-up, since we checked specifically for all the symptom patterns.

Organization and Analysis of Data

We describe below the clinical method on which the findings in this report are based. The systematic method is described, except for the determination of age of onset, in the Appendix.

ADOLESCENT TURMOIL

We realized from the outset that, except in the extremely rare case —that of a previously healthy child in whom symptoms develop at the onset of puberty without any other precipitating factors—it would be difficult to identify adolescent turmoil as the exclusive agent in a psychiatric illness. Adolescent turmoil would probably be only one of a number of identifiable factors precipitating or affecting an illness. Despite the fact that adolescent turmoil was only one of these factors, we considered it sufficient evidence to say that it did play a role in the illness.

We used two evidences of adolescent turmoil. We studied first the age of onset of the present illness, assuming that when it came between eleven and fourteen—that is, in early adolescence—adolescent turmoil was playing a role in the illness. Age of onset was determined by the systematic method. First we defined the present illness as consisting of all those symptoms which brought the patient to the clinic: both the patient's complaints and the symptoms the psychiatrist perceived as related to the complaints. We then defined the duration of present illness as the period of time from the first manifestation of any symptom that was part of the present illness to the date of the interview, even though the symptoms might have had a fluctuating course. Two psychiatrists reviewed every case and, after defining the present illness, made a judgment as to its duration from which they calculated the age of onset. The psychiatrists doing the rating had previously done a test of coding reliability on a random sample of thirty-three cases, in which they had a medium percentage of agreement of 86.5 for duration of illness. When disagreements occurred, they were resolved by joint discussions. This rating had two limitations. Since we took the earliest symptom of the present illness, whether it had a fluctuating course or not, illnesses appeared to have begun at an early age. Also, since it was based on a description of the present illness, it tended to deemphasize underlying character symptomatology. To expand this general notion, we reviewed all the cases, comparing the present clinical picture with the past history and inferring that the presence of newly developed or intensified sexual and aggressive elements in the clinical picture were probably due to adolescent turmoil. The two pieces of evidence, then, consist of age of onset of the illness and a clinical picture containing the elements of conflict known to be associated with this stage in the growth process. It is important to keep in mind that these two pieces of evidence were ascertained differently, the first in a descriptive, systematic manner and the second from a clinical review.

FAMILY RELATIONSHIPS

The material presented is derived from analysis of three interviews, the first conducted by the psychiatrist, the second and third by the social worker. The interviewer, while attempting to get a general evaluation of the psychopathology of the personality of the parent, focused specifically on the attitude of the parent toward the patient. Similar information was obtained from the adolescent. All this material was then reviewed by two social workers under the supervision of the principal investigator to get a final clinical impression.

This combined clinical judgment was based upon both conscious and unconscious aspects of the parent's attitude. The parental attitude was judged to be accepting if it was one of affection for, interest in, and acceptance of the adolescent. It was judged to be pathologic if it was predominantly one of the following: overindulgent, oversolicitous, overprotective, angry, hostile, punitive, restrictive, nagging, sexually provocative, inconsistent, and unable to set limits. When one attitude did not predominate, the parent's attitude was judged to be ambivalent. Of the seventy-two cases reported here, mothers only were seen in fifty-four cases, both parents in fourteen cases, and a parent surrogate in four cases. Consequently, judgments of the father's attitude, based on information obtained from the mother and the adolescent, must be considered relatively unreliable.

Although the material is obviously handicapped by the fact that the parents were seen only once on initial interview, this defect is somewhat mitigated by the glaring quality of the parents' pathology as described in Chapter 4, and also by the fact that the two follow-up interviews by different observers tended to corroborate the initial findings. However, since our study focused more on the adolescent's psychopathology than on the parent's, we shall limit our report of the parents to descriptions of their attitudes.

DIAGNOSTIC DILEMMA

Before taking up the diagnostic dilemma in adolescent psychiatry, it is necessary to consider for a moment the diagnostic dilemma in all of psychiatry.

Some of this dilemma stems from the fact that the present system of classification combines two approaches to diagnosis, the descriptive and the psychodynamic, which have different origins. The former, and historically the earlier, arose from the study of inpatient psychotics when the emphasis was on custodial care. As developed by Kraepelin, it conceived of emotional disorders as disease entities and was descriptive. The latter arose through the study of outpatients where the emphasis was on psychodynamics and treatment. It followed the repudiation of the disease entity concept by Meyer, who then introduced the concept of reaction patterns dependent on constitution and life experiences. Meyer's views were then further elaborated and refined as a result of the profound influence of Freud. The result is a classification system which contains an inherent conceptual conflict in that it is based partly on a disease entity concept and partly a reaction pattern concept. The present system of classification was officially adopted by the American Psychiatric Association in 1917 and then revised in 1933 and 1952. Clearly it still has many pitfalls, which have been well described by Beck [9] as follows: It requires impractically refined distinctions, as in the diagnosis of psychophysiologic reaction as opposed to conversion reaction; it requires unnecessary decisions of weighing, as in judging of predominance between neurotic symptoms and a personality disorder when both are present; and it lacks clear criteria, as in distinguishing certain reactions now labeled schizophrenic from neuroses or schizoid personalities. It has also been attacked for its unreliability, its number of cases left unclassified, and its lack of predictive validity (syndromes of psychosis) [43]. The reliability of psychiatric diagnosis has recently been under study by Beck [7, 8], who reported a higher degree of agreement (54 per cent) on specific diagnoses than had been previously reported. In addition, he reports that when only the major divisions were used (psychosis, neurosis, and character disorder) the degree of agreement was even higher (70 per cent). Though the system has its defects and still requires scientific validation, it is essential for both research and treatment [29, 44].

There are some who would argue that the present system of classification and diagnosis should be discarded, thus perhaps throwing out the baby with the bath water. They apparently misunderstand the purpose of a system of classification, which is to order knowledge in a useful way that can be easily communicated to others. The criterion, then, is not Is it perfect? but Is it useful despite its handicaps? We contend that the present system, though perhaps honored as much in the breach as in the observance, continues to be valuable, not because it places a patient in a neatly compartmented, sterile category, but because it tells us useful things about what is wrong with a patient, what treatment is indicated, and what outcome may be anticipated. These are all not only helpful but indispensable for the clinician in his daily work. I cannot envision that even those who wish to do away with classifications altogether would try to work with patients without at least determining whether a patient had a psychosis, a neurosis, a personality disorder, or an organic disorder. Certainly their dissatisfaction is soundly based, but perhaps a more judicious approach would be to continue to modify the present classification system along more dynamic lines as the increase in knowledge dictates.

Since our focus was on adolescence and not on modification of the existing classification system, we attempted to apply it as currently constructed to our adolescent patients. Our findings are reported primarily for the major divisions (schizophrenia, neurosis, and personality disorder) which have been shown to afford the highest reliability;

in addition, they are based on a five-year history of psychopathology as opposed to a single interview. In studying diagnosis we found, not unexpectedly, that the diagnostic categories as now defined created some difficulties.

Schizophrenia presented the fewest, since it is relatively well defined and readily applicable to the clinical situation.

Psychoneurosis, though also well defined, was more of a problem; the definitions are not so easily applicable to the clinical situation, as is shown by the amount of discussion in the current literature on whether or not a clinical psychoneurosis exists apart from a character neurosis [58]. As discussed in Chapter 9 in more detail, we decided to forgo this differentiation and to use these two terms interchangeably to describe patients whose clinical pictures are similar in that they consist of psychoneurotic symptoms, without schizophrenic or personality disorder pathology, who have neurotic traits in their character structure, and who have a good outcome. We leave to others the issue of whether they represent psychoneuroses or character neuroses. Whichever it is, they are a relatively homogeneous clinical group, significantly different from the other groups.

This brings us to a potpourri of vaguely defined disorders, the personality disorders. The difficulties in the diagnosis of personality disorder are illustrated by the fact that the APA has one classification [2], primarily descriptive in nature, the Veterans Administration has another [57], more dynamically based, and the psychoanalytic literature also has a number of its own [54], including not only those of Freud and his disciples but those of Reich, Horney, and Fromm. Psychoanalysis, now in the phase of developing a comprehensive scheme of characterology, began by stressing the libidinal point of view (zonal phase), emphasizing the erogenous zones as determinants, and postulating oral, anal, phallic, and genital characters. Its second phase stressed the structural concept of the personality (ego, id, superego) and placed character structure in the ego. In addition, other character disorders are described, such as the "as if" and the borderline characters.

In this poorly understood area, the diagnostician finds himself in a maze. He can figuratively pay his money and take his choice, for each classification has its strengths and weaknesses. We finally decided to use the classification in the APA manual despite its limitations. Though mainly descriptive and often vague, it allows us to spell out clearly what we mean by a given diagnosis, and being the most widely accepted it offers a broad base for comparison with others.

In using the classification we encountered a number of obvious roadblocks that, as this area is studied more clearly, might well be taken into account in future revisions. For example, there was no provision for sexual perversions except in the sociopathic personality, and a number of our patients had perversions without being sociopathic. Further, except for compulsive personality disorder, there was no provision for patients with neurotic character disorders in the psychoanalytic sense of the term. Moreover, the clinical picture or outcome of the patients with compulsive personality disorder resembled more closely those with a neurotic character disorder than those with a personality disorder as the APA uses the term.

Let us now consider how we applied this system of classification. It was our purpose to approximate the usual clinical situation, in which the psychiatrist, seeing the patient at one point in time, must do his evaluation on the basis of a cross section. Accordingly, after the systematic analysis had been finished, we turned again to the basic material in the charts and first reviewed only the initial interview to arrive at a differential diagnosis, spelling out the evidence for each of the differential possibilities and thus pointing up the unresolved diagnostic problems. Then we added the vantage point of time (five years) to the usual clinical cross section by tracing the diagnostic developments through two follow-up interviews until the patient was at least chronologically past adolescence, spelling out how the diagnostic problems were resolved and also what remained unresolved.

There were some methodologic handicaps. Initially the patients were seen only once, although by two psychiatrists. The purpose was to approximate a relatively rapid psychiatric evaluation, which often has to be done on the basis of a somewhat cursory interview rather than an intensive one. There were no psychological tests. In retrospect, these are a handicap to the delineation of diagnostic problems, since often a number of interviews are required, as well as psychological testing, to get enough information to have confidence in a diagnosis. However, it is pertinent to mention here that in many cases the diagnosis was quite clear at this level of study, and in some others seen in treatment up to a year, the diagnosis, when in doubt, did not become clear but remained uncertain until three or four years had passed. In addition, it is not uncommon in clinical experience to find that when the clinician is in doubt the findings of the psychological test are often also equivocal. Nevertheless, we may here paraphrase the words of a very experienced researcher: "If we had it to do over again, we'd do it differently." Lastly, although we only saw the patients once initially, we do have two follow-up interviews spread over a period of five years to fortify our final diagnostic judgment.

OUTCOME

After many trials at subdividing the APA concept of impairment of functioning into specifically defined subsidiary elements—such as impairment at school, in social life, in relationships with parents—we were unsatisfied because, although these categories might tell us much about school functioning or about social functioning for the whole group, they told us almost nothing about their relationships in the individual patient. We finally decided that the APA concept was still the most effective and most appropriate, since it took into account all of these factors operating in the individual patient. All the material in each case, therefore, was evaluated by the psychiatrist, who used his clinical judgment to rate the level of impairment of functioning on follow-up thus: minimal, 0–10 per cent; mild, 20–30 per cent; moderate, 30–50 per cent; severe, over 50 per cent. Though this is admittedly a gross rating and open to individual bias, it still gives greatest weight to all the factors operating at the same time and uses the best instrument for its measurement—the psychiatrist's judgment. Although someone else reviewing these patients might place one or another at a different level of impairment of functioning, my supposition is that the majority would end up at the same levels of impairment.

Certainly this approach, as illustrated in Chapter 12, did help to significantly differentiate the patient's levels of functioning one from the other. While defining impairment in terms of functioning is adequate for most purposes, as we know from psychoanalysis, it leaves something to be desired, since often patients (obsessive-compulsives, for example) do learn to function well but at the cost of rather than through the expression of their inner emotional needs. We would, therefore, like to know more about these patients. If impairment is now defined not in terms of functioning, but in terms of underlying conflicts with regard to dependency needs, to sexual drives, and to aggressive impulses, we want to know to what extent the patients have made some comfortable resolution of conflicts in these three key areas.

We also want to know to what extent, in the course of the resolution, their character structure remained free from psychopathologic traits, thereby enabling the diverse elements of their mental apparatus to blend harmoniously to produce self-actualization or optimal functioning. Unfortunately this study was not designed to elicit such data since it is based on three interviews only with patient and mother over a five-year period. Nevertheless, it would be shortsighted indeed not to utilize the material we do have to make what contribution we can, keeping in mind that it is at best impressionistic.

We again reviewed, from this point of view, the twenty-seven patients minimally impaired, assuming that in the others the presence of more than mild impairment was evidence of their inability to resolve the conflicts. In this review we used the following manifestations as evidence of unresolved dependency needs: need to be cared for; excessive need for approval, with anxiety when it is not forthcoming; clinging to a parent; and difficulty in acting independently and establishing dependency relationships with persons other than parents. Evidence for conflicts with aggressive impulses consisted of such things as inability to express anger freely or without great anxiety and guilt; handling it by suppression, acting-out, or withdrawal; and difficulties with self-assertion. Conflicts about sexual impulses presented more of a problem. Although sometimes the evidence of conflicts was quite clear, where it was not clear it was often impossible to probe with sufficient depth in one interview to get the necessary information. We therefore decided to take advantage of the information that was consistent and reliable by noting whether the patient had had at least one emotional involvement with a member of the opposite sex and also whether he had had sexual intercourse. It seemed fair to assume that someone who had not had one close relationship with the opposite sex by the time he was twenty-one had difficulties in this area. Sexual intercourse, though not a reliable guide as to the presence or absence of sexual conflicts, at least told us that the patient's sexual development had progressed this far.

TREATMENT

During the five-year follow-up period thirty-eight patients received outpatient treatment, eleven received inpatient treatment, and thirty-one received no treatment. Fourteen patients were treated for less than six months, nine patients for six to twelve months, and twenty-one for more than a year. The same problem exists here as we had with the study of underlying conflicts: this study was not designed to evaluate psychiatric treatment. However, again as was the case with underlying conflicts, we do have some information which, while not part of the research project itself, may contribute to the question of the effect of treatment. Forty-two patients received psychotherapy, thirty at the Payne Whitney Clinic.

We reviewed the entire treatment record, in some cases of three or four years' duration, to answer three questions: Did the patient improve under psychiatric treatment? If so, how did psychiatric treatment help? If it did not help, why not? One final caution: The clinical material on treatment had certain limitations that it would be well to keep in mind before considering the findings. First, this was a retrospective view; treatment was studied after the fact rather than as an ongoing process. Second, since the course and results of treatment were not a planned part of the research project, patient records prepared by psychiatrists not involved in the research generally lacked detailed reports of the patient's content of mood, thought, and behavior and included very little of the psychiatrist's therapeutic activity. Therefore, the best we can do is get an impression of the recurrent themes discussed, and ascertain whether or not the patient improved.

A few words about the type of psychiatric treatment and its duration and frequency are pertinent. The patients were seen in psychotherapy by a third-year resident psychiatrist once a week and the mothers by a social worker once a week. The duration of treatment varied from a few weeks to, in some cases, three to six years. The therapeutic approach could be described as eclectic. It stressed psychoanalytic theory for the understanding of dynamics, but therapeutic activity was directive and supportive, in an attempt to provide a source of identification for the patient and alternate means of handling his emotional conflicts. The resident and the social worker were seen weekly in supervision, a number by the author, who found that to review one's supervisory notes eight years later and wiser is an instructive process.

SYMPTOM FLUCTUATIONS

Since symptomatology can theoretically shift within an hour or a day, as well as over longer periods, the best evidence for variation in symptom pattern would be that derived from patients seen frequently in treatment over a long time. This procedure permits observations of sudden transient shifts in symptomatology which might be missed by having interviews spaced at greater intervals. The complexity of the problem is indicated by the fact that even under these circumstances it is necessary to account for the effect of treatment on the observed shift in symptom patterns.

All the patients were interviewed three times: initially at the age of sixteen, two and a half years later at eighteen and a half, and five years later at twenty-one—the chronological end of adolescence. Our findings can be viewed, therefore, as three cross sections at three points in time, rather than as a continuous record derived from a treatment setting. However, as mentioned, thirty of the seventy-two patients were also seen in treatment, and our retrospective analysis of the records of those thirty supported the findings presented. This material was not included here because it was not a part of the research methodology. Beginning with the coded symptom patterns, we clinically reviewed the cases by diagnostic category throughout the three interviews to determine which symptom patterns persisted and which dropped out.

SECTION II
DYNAMIC FACTORS

CHAPTER 3

ADOLESCENT TURMOIL

> For every youth and maiden who is not strictly se
> cluded or very stupid, adolescence is a period of dis-
> tressful perplexity, of hidden hypothesis, misunder-
> stood hints, checked urgency, and wild stampedes of
> the imagination.
> —H. G. Wells: *Joan and Peter*

ADOLESCENCE HAS BEEN STUDIED from many points of view. For example, the anthropologist or sociologist looking at it as a period in the life cycle of the race—a time span, stretching from puberty to an ill-defined point called maturity—has studied its social and cultural manifestations. Our own interest is in adolescence as a stage in individual growth and development which has been notorious throughout the centuries as one of great emotional upset with wide fluctuations in behavior. This stage, initiated by the biologic event of puberty, is characterized not only by physical changes but by profound consequences for emotional life. The events of puberty enhance all instinctual drives, notably the sexual and the aggressive, and result in the initiation of emotional conflicts as well as exacerbation of all those previously unresolved. Further complications are the needs that soon arise to accomplish certain growth tasks, such as emancipation from dependency and assumption of a heterosexual role as the adolescent moves toward maturity. The emotional vicissitudes involved in dealing with these intra- and extrapsychic tensions inherent in the growth process are what we define as *adolescent turmoil.*

Our purpose is to describe the relationships of adolescent turmoil to psychiatric illness. Is it incidental to psychiatric illness? Does it initiate psychiatric illness in previously healthy children? Does it intensify illnesses which have been carried over from childhood? Or does it perhaps exacerbate childhood illnesses that have been in remission?

Of the seventy-two patients, fifty-three showed evidence that adolescent turmoil affected their illness. Of these, thirty-one had both an onset between ages eleven and fourteen and sexual or aggressive elements in their clinical picture, and twenty-two, whose illnesses began either earlier or later, showed primarily sexual and aggressive elements in their clinical picture. In ten of the remaining nineteen, the clinical picture was that of a chronic, severe personality disorder, or schizophrenia that began early in life and followed a course little influenced by adolescence; in seven the data were not clear enough to come to a conclusion; and in two with character neurosis, adolescent turmoil seemed irrelevant to the clinical picture.

Table 2.   Age of Onset of Present Illness by Diagnosis

Age of Onset	Diagnosis		
	Schizophrenia	Personality Disorder	Character Neurosis
15 and over	3 (16.6%)	6 (14.0%)	2 (18.2%)
11–14	5 (27.7%)	20 (46.5%)	6 (54.5%)
7–10	2 (11.1%)	8 (18.6%)	2 (18.2%)
Before 7	8 (44.4%)	9 (20.9%)	1 (9.1%)
Total	18	43	11

Table 2 shows that in 55.5 per cent of those with schizophrenia their illness began at the age of ten or before, and in about 28 per cent it began between the ages of eleven and fourteen. Personality disorder first appeared in fewer at the age of ten or before (39.5 per cent) and in more between eleven and fourteen (46.5 per cent). Those with character neurosis show an almost opposite picture from those with schizophrenia: In only about 27 per cent did the illness have its onset before adolescence, and in 54.5 per cent it started during early adolescence. These findings indicate that, in terms of the age when a clinical illness begins, adolescent turmoil exerts its most pronounced effect on a character neurosis, a pronounced but somewhat lesser effect in personality disorders, and a still smaller effect in schizophrenia, since the latter illness had begun long before adolescence in over half these patients. As mentioned previously, the findings for personality disorder, based on a description of present illness, contain an artifact, for this rating omitted the most essential component of a personality disorder—a past history of underlying character traits (see Chapter 2). We shall describe later how a more detailed clinical study of cases of personality disorder extends the findings.

Let us now consider each diagnostic category in more clinical detail.

Schizophrenia

The major theme, in eight patients, was the intensification or exacerbation of a childhood schizophrenia which, in some cases, had manifested itself in childhood as a conduct disorder. Following are several examples: A fifteen-year-old girl was diagnosed and treated for childhood schizophrenia at the age of five, with symptoms of mutism, withdrawal, social isolation, and restlessness. She showed a temporary remission, but after menarche she became sexually preoccupied, her aggressiveness increased to the point where she was destructive and assaultive, she suffered periods of excitement and depression, and she began sexual acting-out. This is a dramatic instance of one way the clinical picture of schizophrenia is colored by the pressures of the adolescent growth process; withdrawn and isolated since age five, the girl began with the onset of menses to act-out, both aggressively and sexually. However, though the most dramatic, it is not the most representative example, since the more common picture was not reversal but intensification of preexistent symptoms. In another case, a fifteen-year-old boy, with clear evidence of a schizophrenic reaction, a lifelong history of marked anxiety and tension, and a thinking disorder, had great difficulty in school. At thirteen his anxiety and tension increased, his socialization decreased to the point of isolation, and he became more hostile and defiant with his mother. Finally, an example of the exacerbation of a schizophrenic process which had manifested itself as a conduct disorder in childhood: A seventeen-year-old girl, with a history of conduct disorder, anxiety, and obesity throughout childhood, under the pressure of sexual preoccupations experienced an increase in her anxiety and became depressed.

The two remaining themes are revealed in the following: In three cases adolescent turmoil was seemingly unrelated to a chronic schizophrenic process beginning early in childhood and showing a course of progressive deterioration throughout adolescence. In two cases turmoil was associated with the acute onset of a schizophrenic condition in patients with no past history of difficulty. In five cases the data were not clear enough to warrant a conclusion.

To summarize then, adolescent turmoil affects schizophrenia in a number of ways. The most common theme is intensification or exacerbation of a childhood chronic schizophrenia. Second is the seeming initiation of an acute schizophrenic process without a past history of difficulty, and third is a chronic deteriorating schizophrenia in which adolescent turmoil seems to have no part.

Personality Disorder

In thirty-one of the forty-three patients with personality disorder we found turmoil related to a clinical exacerbation of a long-standing personality disorder—in seven of the ten sociopaths, fifteen of the twenty passive-aggressives, five of the eight miscellaneous, and four of the five epileptics. The sociopaths revealed two major themes: first, aggression manifested early in childhood as conduct disorder, which later in adolescence became intensified, with flagrant acting-out to the point of antisocial behavior; second, a history of neurotic symptoms and conduct disorder in childhood, both of which became intensified in adolescence.

The first theme was evident in a sixteen-and-a-half-year-old boy who since early childhood had expressed aggression passively by procrastination and avoidance of responsibility and actively by temper tantrums and difficulty in controlling his impulses. His symptoms had also included lying, nail-biting, and thumb-sucking. At thirteen he started to have more conflict with his nagging mother, became depressed, and began to steal and engage in other delinquent activities. The second theme was illustrated in a fifteen-and-a-half-year-old boy with a low IQ and a childhood history of anxiety, nightmares, and stuttering. He was also self-centered, passively rebellious, and doing poorly in school. At the onset of adolescence he became more anxious and more openly rebellious by refusing to go to school and was finally arrested by the police for carrying a gun.

Those in the diagnostic category of passive-aggressive showed a major theme of increased conflict at home accompanied by withdrawal, plus an increase in anxiety, depression, and/or psychoneurotic symptoms. In few was there a rise in the overt expression of aggression. Several were conspicuously preoccupied with masturbation and/or perversions. Two examples follow. A seventeen-year-old boy had a past history of enuresis till the age of seven, clinging to his mother when the father was away for a year, and marginal schoolwork. At the age of thirteen, when the mother was operated on for cancer of the breast, he developed marked anxiety, tension, nervousness, lack of interest in school, temper tantrums, compulsive ruminations, concentration difficulty, and severe accident proneness to the extent of suffering a number of broken bones within a very short time. Another seventeen-year-old boy had a childhood history of difficulty in social adjustment and enuresis which persisted till he was fifteen. At age twelve, after his father died, and with the onset of puberty at age thirteen in the setting of living with his sexually promiscuous and provocative mother, he withdrew further from social activity and had no friends of either sex. He masturbated frequently with guilt feelings and voyeuristic fantasies. Finally, at the age of seventeen, he began to act these fantasies out and was arrested as a peeping tom.

In epileptics, who will be considered in more detail later as a separate group, a common theme was increased aggression, which brought them into greater conflict with their parents and produced a depression.

Character Neurosis

Of the eleven patients with character neurosis showing evidence that adolescent turmoil played a role in their illness, nine were almost evenly divided between two themes: first, acute onset of symptoms in early adolescence without a prior history of difficulty, and second, exacerbation of past symptoms, also early in adolescence.

In the first group, four patients developed conversion symptoms, two girls having abdominal pain after the onset of menses, and one girl, age fourteen, having severe conversion symptoms after her boy friend had raped her. A boy developed hysterical, convulsive-like seizures which appeared to be defenses against his hostile impulses. The fifth patient of this group was brought to the clinic for engaging in homosexual play.

In the second group, two girls had past histories of compulsive character structure. One, following menarche at age nine, developed anxiety whenever in mixed company; this was followed by a depression at age fourteen, when she was rejected by her boy friend. The other, at age twelve and a half, following the death of her father, developed a severe depression. A boy aged thirteen and a half, with a past history of asthma, in the setting of living alone with his mother and having a possibly homosexual brother, developed marked anxiety, tension, concentration difficulty, and insomnia; his usually excellent school functioning declined, and he became preoccupied with being a homosexual. The last, a girl of seventeen, had a past history from age five to eleven of vomiting when excited. She had her menarche at age eleven; and on her first date, at age fourteen, developed anxiety, nervousness, vomiting, chills, and excessive jealousy about her boy friend.

The clinical picture of these patients with character neurosis seems clearly in contrast to that of the patients with personality disorder and schizophrenia. Half had only mild and circumscribed previous difficulties, and indeed half of the psychoneurotics gave no such history, so that one cannot escape the impression that the beginning of adolescence did bring on a dramatic change, particularly in those with severe conversion symptoms. As we shall see in Chapter 11, despite the fact that the psychoneurotic illnesses were severe on admission, the outcome was good. Those with personality disorder and schizophrenia, on the other hand, showed more of a direct connection between their early childhood developmental problems and their clinical picture in adolescence.

Considering now the question to which this chapter was addressed, we find that the relationships of adolescent turmoil to psychiatric illness vary somewhat by type of illness. Although in two patients with schizophrenia and five with psychoneurosis, adolescent turmoil apparently brought on a clinical illness in the absence of prior psychopathology, in a far greater number (forty-four) it seemed to exacerbate and give its own particular coloring to previously existent psychopathology. In those who were schizophrenic, adolescent turmoil tended to cause further deterioration of a chronic illness or to exacerbate one that had been in remission. Occasionally there was a reversal from withdrawal to acting-out symptomatology, but more usual was the intensification of preexistent symptoms. In the personality disorders, adolescent turmoil invariably exacerbated long-standing personality problems. Among the sociopaths, preexistent difficulties with the expression of aggression, as shown by conduct disorders, markedly intensified, with acting-out becoming more flagrant and frequently antisocial. On the other hand, those with passive-aggressive personality disorders usually experienced more of an intensification of anxiety, depression, and psychoneurotic symptoms; acting-out was less frequent, preoccupation with sexual perversions more common. Lastly, in the character neurosis group, adolescent turmoil tended to precipitate an acute clinical illness, either in a patient without previous history of difficulty or in one who had had only mild and circumscribed neurotic symptoms or a neurotic character structure.

CHAPTER 4

PARENTAL ATTITUDES AND FAMILY RELATIONSHIPS

> Do ye hear the children weeping, O my brothers,
> Ere the sorrow comes with years?
> The child's sob in the silence curses deeper
> Than the strong man in his wrath.
> —Elizabeth B. Browning: "The
> Cry of the Children"

THIS CHAPTER, dealing with the role the parents play in the adolescent's psychiatric illness, is addressed to such questions as: How pathologic are the parents' attitudes? Do they tend to be interested, accepting, and supporting, or disinterested, rejecting, and destructive? Can we generalize as to the relationship of parental attitude to the pathologic behavior of the adolescent? How much conflict is there between parent and adolescent? Is it about adolescent issues, such as emancipation, peer relationships, and sexual behavior, or has it been carried over from childhood, revolving around, for example, unresolved dependency needs or poorly developed ego controls?

The attitudes of the parents of the adolescents in the personality disorder and schizophrenia categories differed dramatically from the attitudes of the parents in the character neurosis category. There was not a single adolescent in the two former categories who did not have at least one parent with a pathologic attitude. In addition, the parent with the flagrant pathologic attitude was the predominant influence in the family, while the other parent, whose attitude was usually somewhat accepting, tended to play a minor role and to have little influence on the adolescent. For the patients in the character neurosis category, however, not only did fewer parents have pathologic attitudes, but, as was not the case in the other two categories, where one parent had a pathologic attitude, the other seemed to show enough concern, interest, and affection to modify the effect of the pathologic attitude on the adolescent. There was such variety in the patterns of parental attitudes that it was not possible to generalize regarding their relationship to the pathologic behavior of the adolescent except in the personality disorder subgroups of passive-aggressive disorders, which we shall consider in more detail later. Finally, some conflict between parent and adolescent was present in most cases, though again it was less in the character neurosis category than in the schizophrenia and personality disorder categories. This conflict was most often related to long-standing pathologic attitudes of both parent and adolescent that had predated adolescence.

There is another conclusion which, though quite striking in itself, is less reliable because it has to be inferred from the descriptive information about attitudes of fathers as obtained from the adolescents and their mothers. The fathers of adolescents in the schizophrenia and personality disorder categories played an inadequate role because they were either absent from the home, uninterested in their adolescent, psychiatrically ill themselves, or excluded from the family by a domineering mother.

Let us now take up in more detail the parental attitudes under each diagnostic category.

Schizophrenia

The most common theme, found in fourteen of the eighteen cases, was that one parent had a pathologic attitude (in ten cases the mother; in four cases the father) while the other was either psychiatrically ill, or distant and uninterested in the adolescent, or, even though relatively accepting in attitude, played too minimal a role in the family to counteract the influence of the predominant parent. For two other adolescents both parents' attitudes were pathologic, and for the remaining two we were unable to make a conclusive judgment. Since there was such wide variety among the specific pathologic attitudes, we will describe a few in general terms and illustrate two in more clinical detail.

One mother, diagnosed as having a hysterical personality disorder with schizoid trends, although she had some basic understanding of and affection for her son, related to him as a peer and hence was flirtatious and sexually provocative toward him. Her compulsive need for male attention, however, led her to the point of physical neglect of her son more often than to exhibiting this pathologic attitude. The father, diagnosed as a sociopath, was divorced from the mother, and although he too expressed some affectionate feelings for his son, he was so irresponsible in his role of father that he neglected and even ignored the boy.

In another family the mother was ambitious for her son but was distant, unaffectionate, domineering, and demanding. She parceled out acceptance and love in proportion to her son's achievement according to her standards. The father had died when the patient was five, and although more accepting of the child, he had been a passive, quiet man, dominated by his aggressive wife to such an extent that he had little early influence on his son, who at the age of sixteen found it difficult to remember him at all.

In a third family the mother, diagnosed as having a schizophrenic illness, was grossly overprotective, continued to treat her son as a young child, and was unaware of his adolescent problems. The father was emotionally cold and distant but, unlike most of the fathers, professed and openly manifested an interest in his son by having some companionable relationship with him.

In a fourth family the mother, diagnosed as having a psychoneurosis, was tense, explosive, domineering, and overwhelmed with the responsibilities of being a mother. While she showed some affection for her daughter, she was unable to comprehend or respond to her needs. The father was separated from this family. He was reported to lack interest in the patient and rarely saw her.

In the four families in which the father had the pathologic attitude, he tended to be critical, domineering, hot tempered, and explosive. Three of the fathers were also essentially cold and distant and without affection for, or interest in, the patient. On the other hand, the mothers in these four families played passive roles in their relationships with their husbands and children and were seemingly without insight into the problems of the patient.

The adolescents in these eighteen families tended to be resentful and hostile toward the parent with the pathologic attitude and relatively at ease with the opposite parent. Most of them were outspoken about their hostility, while four, all of whom experienced extreme rejection by one or both parents, tended to deny being resentful. With several exceptions, overt conflict was present between the parents and the adolescent. It was conflict, however, that had existed long prior to adolescence and was seemingly related to the symptomatology of the patient's illness and the parent's pathologic attitude and not to the problems of adolescent turmoil such as the struggle for emancipation, peer relationships, or sexual behavior. We illustrate these themes in more detail below:

A fourteen-year-old boy, in the ninth grade, gave a history of having been in overt conflict with his mother since the age of five. He had difficulty because of his poor conduct in school, which was manifested by anxiety, restlessness, and attention-getting behavior. He also had temper outbursts and behaved destructively in his home. The father was chronically ill, was generally removed from the children, and, although he had some interest in the patient, had had no understanding of or ability to cope with his behavior. Recently the patient had begun to question his mother regarding masturbation and sexual intercourse. The mother, an infantile, nagging, psychoneurotic woman with ulcerative colitis, was pathologically dependent on the patient, sexually provocative with him, and unable to discipline him. She was indecisive, inconsistent, possessive, and too fearful of losing her son to set limits for his behavior. This immature boy with poor control of sexual and aggressive impulses, on the other hand, was bound by his pathologic dependency to his mother, frightened by her seductive behavior, and markedly ambivalent about her. The two were locked in a mutually provocative and sadomasochistic relationship in which the patient acted-out his hostility by disobedience, arguing, refusing to help around the house, and occasionally actually becoming destructive. This is a representative example of a mother with a pathologic attitude, an inadequate father, and long-standing conflict originating in childhood. Clearly, adolescent problems, as indicated by the patient's concern about sexual matters, were present, but secondary to the persistent and chronic differences with the mother.

The next case illustrates the occurrence of the pathologic attitude in the father.

The patient, a sixteen-year-old boy, was referred to the clinic because of failures over many years and social difficulty of lifelong duration. He was very shy and had few friends. He also had had a fear of bathrobes since the age of two when his grandfather died and he had a tonsillectomy. The father was critical, demanding, unsympathetic, and totally lacking in understanding of the patient's illness. He was critical of his son's lifelong shyness and taunted him about his fears. He resented the boy's lack of response to his efforts to teach him to be more aggressive and outgoing. He put continual pressure on the boy with his nagging demands and reacted to the patient's symptoms with anger and explosions of temper. The son responded to his father's anger and pressure by withdrawing, which only provoked the father more. The mother, on the other hand, though she showed some interest in her son, played a submissive role to the dominant father. The patient would complain to the mother about his father but would keep silent and slink away whenever the father was around. He seemed to enjoy finding fault with him to his mother, and in the clinic as well, and expressed a delusional fear that the father "smoked a cigar to harm him." Clearly the conflict here stemmed from a long-standing pathologic attitude of rejection on the part of the father, who had never been able to understand and therefore meet the needs of a seriously ill child. The child in turn reacted with dependency on the mother and withdrawal from the father, the latter constantly provoked afresh to demands for a show of aggressiveness in his shy and fearful son.

Personality Disorder

Here again, as in the schizophrenia category, the common theme was that of one parent with a pathologic attitude, most often the mother. The father typically had little interest in or influence over child rearing, though attitudes among the forty-two fathers ranged from lack of interest, irresponsibility, and passivity to possessiveness and demandingness. Although the patterns of parental attitudes varied widely, an exception was apparent in the subcategory of passive-aggressive, where in contrast to the other subcategories of this group there was a uniformity of parental attitude that seemed to be related to the pathologic behavior of the patient. Here we found, for fourteen out of nineteen, an aggressive, domineering mother and a passively rebellious adolescent. In these same fourteen cases, with the mother aggressive and domineering, two fathers were absent from the home and twelve were quite passive. Seven of the latter were both distant and uninterested, leaving only five who were essentially passive but who did show some interest in their adolescent.

Again, as was seen in those with schizophrenia, the adolescent with personality disorder was resentful and ambivalent toward the parent with the pathologic attitude and had some acceptance of the other parent. Six patients showed a surprising degree of awareness of their family conflict, verbalizing quite freely their desire for closeness with the parent, as well as their awareness of and resentment about parental rejection. Overt conflict was exhibited by all but one or two of these adolescents. It began early in childhood in all but two and in most instances was specifically related to the acting-out behavior of the adolescent. We present four case illustrations. The first two are from the sociopathic subcategory.

A fourteen-year-old boy, diagnosed as a sociopath, gave a history since the age of five of anxiety, with insomnia, restlessness, and concentration difficulty. Although he made passing grades in school, he complained of being bored, restless, and unable to do his schoolwork. He was overtalkative and exhibited other attention-getting behavior in school. At age thirteen and a half, following the onset of an acute mastitis and starting in at a new school, his anxiety increased, he came into increasing conflict with his parents, and he began to fail in his schoolwork. He experienced intense rivalry toward his sister, whom he believed his father preferred. He had depressive thoughts, often of running away, whenever he was punished by his mother.

The mother was overindulgent on the one hand, getting the patient out of bed in the morning and pampering him with solicitous attentions, but on the other hand she was sexually provocative and called him a fag and a fairy. In addition, she was obsessively preoccupied with his behavior; especially when he stayed out late at night, or was otherwise disobedient, she became unduly punitive and restrictive. The patient related that there were books on homosexuality around the house which he was not permitted to read. His conflict with his mother revolved around stealing of money, the time he came in at night, his schoolwork, his responsibilities at home, and his behavior with his sister.

The father, who was rather emphatically distant and disinterested in the children, had a family history of one sister who committed suicide and another who was currently institutionalized in a mental hospital. Although essentially disinterested, he was at the same time severely critical and would barge into the patient's room to hit him when he misbehaved. He also demanded that the children wait on him and obey him instantly.

The patient had a history of masturbation, beginning in childhood and continuing to the time of the interview. The mother's ambivalence was indicated by her comment "It's all right unless I catch you" to her son about this behavior. The patient's acting-out behavior clearly seemed to be related to a deep-seated sense of guilt and to an expression of his rage at the mother and the father, thereby provoking retribution in the form of punishment.

A fifteen-year-old girl had a childhood history of being a feeding problem and of soiling until age two and a half. She was a highly emotional, tense child with feelings of inferiority, temper tantrums, nail-biting, thumb-sucking, and asthma until age ten. Since the onset of adolescence, she had had recurrent episodes of depression and elation, expressing a good deal of profanity. She had been a truant from school and was in intense conflict with her mother. She came to the clinic with a depression, having made a suicidal gesture following rejection by a boy.

The mother and father had been divorced five years prior to the interview. The mother was an infantile, narcissistic, dependent woman, whose life was run for her by her own mother. She was quite openly hostile to and rejecting of the patient and so preoccupied with her own problems and her quarrels with her divorced husband that she had no time for the patient. She was herself sexually preoccupied, probably sexually promiscuous, and overly suspicious of the patient's sexual activities, perhaps provoking her by her inferences. Since the divorce the father had also shown little interest in the patient, the mother turning the patient against the father.

The next two case studies illustrate personality disorder of the passive-aggressive type.

A fourteen-year-old boy gave a four-year history, following the birth of his first sibling in the mother's second marriage, of rebellion and disobedience toward the mother, hostility toward the sibling, soiling at home but not at school or at play, stealing from markets, and failing at school. The mother was rigid, compulsive, and perfectionistic. With the patient she was domineering, hostile, rejecting, controlling, and in turn overwhelmed by the patient's hostility. At times she was able to understand his difficulties, but they more often provoked hostility in her. She had no awareness of her own involvement in his problems. She was able to give affection only when the patient conformed to her own rigid standards of behavior. She and the patient's father had been divorced when the patient was three, until which time the father had been active in the patient's upbringing, but afterwards he had little to do with him and became disinterested and totally rejecting. At first the stepfather was friendly and made an effort to take some interest in the patient but was generally passive and uninvolved with him. After his own first child was born what little interest he had quickly waned.

A thirteen-and-a-half-year-old boy with a passive-aggressive disorder was brought to the clinic by his domineering mother. She complained of her son's school difficulties, although he was passing in all his studies. She also complained that he was overcompliant, forgetful, immature, unassertive, and afraid of authority. The mother considered herself a "horrible" unpleasant woman, with a bad disposition. She was hostile, tense, perfectionistic, depressed, irritable, critical, a worrier, without friends or social life.

She and the quiet, withdrawn, "pleasant" father had been divorced when the patient was four. She and the stepfather, an even-tempered man who "lets things slide by," had an apparently satisfactory relationship. Her attitude toward the patient evidenced lack of interest during his early childhood, when she more or less abandoned him to his paternal grandparents until he was eleven. This action was due in part to the mother's physical illness with tuberculosis, but the arrangement was maintained long after it was necessary despite the patient's obvious preference for his mother. Her relationship with the patient was consequently severely conflict and guilt ridden. She was punitive, rejecting, demanding, hostile, and always angry—particularly at his reaction to her, i.e., his overcompliance, passivity, and mild acting-out in school. She was aware of her attitudes but unable to do anything about them. The patient reported, however, that his mother could be affectionate with him at times.

The father was apparently basically accepting with his son when in contact with him, but he lacked interest and contact was infrequent. The stepfather was, however, interested in the patient, was not critical, and tried to influence the mother to handle the child differently, though without much success.

These four cases illustrate clearly the theme of one parent with a pathologic attitude, usually the mother, while the other parent played a less active role in the family. In addition, they show that conflict had existed from early childhood and was in origin unrelated to, although perhaps accentuated by, issues having to do with adolescence.

Character Neurosis

The parental attitudes toward the eleven adolescents with character neurosis differed dramatically from those of the parents in the diagnostic categories described above. In five cases both parents were found to have accepting, interested attitudes, and in five more, although one parent had a pathologic attitude, the other was predominantly accepting. There was only one case with pathologic attitude in both parents.

The common theme in eight of the eleven mothers was an attitude of acceptance, warmth, affection, interest, and understanding. This is not to say that their attitudes contained no pathologic elements. For example, some parents had inordinately high expectations for conformity or achievement, usually manifested in covert pressures going beyond the limits of support and encouragement. Others were overprotective and overindulgent. There was also some lack of insight and a tendency to criticize and to withhold approval for any achievement the child might have made. However, the predominance of warmth, interest, and concern served as a protection against these negative facets.

Seven fathers had mostly accepting attitudes, while five had pathologic attitudes. The accepting fathers, unlike the fathers of patients with schizophrenia and personality disorder, were considerably involved in the responsibilities of child rearing and were not just good-natured, passive figures on the sidelines. Marriages, moreover, tended to be stable. In only two were the mothers characterized as the dominant partners; the fathers were warm, affectionate, interested, and close—two of them to the point of mild overindulgence. Although the pathologic attitudes of the five fathers varied and there were some elements of passive disinterest as seen in other diagnostic categories, we did not find, except in one case, that almost total passive rejection noted in the fathers in the other categories. For the most part, in this category of character neurosis, pathologic attitudes of the fathers were evidenced in their being irritable, tense, and critical and in two cases physically abusive when drunk. We see a further difference from the other diagnostic categories in the degree of conflict and in the attitudes of the adolescents themselves. In seven cases overt conflict was never an issue, while in five some conflict with one or both parents was described. When the parent had predominantly positive feelings, so did the patient. When the father's attitude was pathologic, the patient's responses came to be avoidance and disinterest. The following case illustrates these themes.

A sixteen-year-old girl, in the eleventh grade, had a past history of being extremely competitive, perfectionistic, and successful in school. From the age of eleven to the time of the interview she had experienced an increasingly acute anxiety in mixed company and for the past two years feelings of inadequacy and depression following rejection by her boy friend. She had avoided dating situations with boys, her school performance had mildly decreased in excellence, and she finally decided to stay home from school for a week because she was "not prepared." The diagnostic impression was anxiety and depression in the setting of a compulsive character disorder. The mother was a compulsive, controlling, intelligent, capable woman, who tended to intellectualize her feelings and could not admit feelings without a covering rationalization. She wanted to be a perfect parent of a perfect child. She found it hard to accept the dependency needs and other manifestations of immaturity in the patient. She was far too controlling in her discipline and unaware of the hidden pressures for achievement which her daughter felt. At the same time she was warmly interested in, and genuinely concerned about, her daughter and wanted to gain an understanding of her problems. Although he was a quiet, shy, interested, passive, unassertive man, the father was nevertheless actively interested in the patient and in her upbringing.

Let us return now to the questions to which this chapter was addressed and recapitulate first, in general terms, the findings for the schizophrenia and personality disorder diagnostic categories. For these two categories one gets the overwhelming impression of parents who are ill themselves, many with schizophrenia or a personality disorder, and whose illness seems to manifest itself prominently in their relationships with their children. Unable to cope with their own lives effectively, they find the intrusion of children with their dependency needs an added strain which they tolerate only with great difficulty. Conflict begins early in life and revolves around very basic childhood issues. It is made increasingly grave for the child by parental inability to face the burden of his dependency needs and by parental inconsistency in disciplinary measures and in setting limits to behavior. These pathologic attitudes often reach the proportions of outright neglect and rejection of all responsibilities of parenthood, with resultant destructive effects on the personality structure of the child.

Thus the adolescent is placed in a particularly serious "bind" since he enters adolescence and the renewed struggle with his maturing sexual and aggressive instincts hindered by unresolved childhood conflicts. He is compelled, figuratively speaking, to get in and fight the battle of his adolescence with one hand tied behind his back. That is, if his childhood years have not taught him control of impulses, how can he learn control when these impulses are newly reinforced? How can he, at this time of life, turn to his parents for support in the battle? Having failed in his childhood in their task of providing affection and control, they are now extremely poor sources of identification for their struggling adolescent. Adolescence, then, for these patients seems to be mostly both a persistence and a renewal of childhood conflicts rather than a fresh grappling with growth problems of the adolescent years. Consequently, in those with schizophrenia and personality disorder conflicts persist from childhood and confuse and aggravate adolescent issues such as the struggle for emancipation, preoccupation with sex, and competition to establish their place with their peers.

Turning to adolescents in the diagnostic category of character neurosis, we find a much more optimistic picture. Not only are the parents healthier, but when one parent has a pathologic attitude, the other counters it through a positive and healthy attitude. The adolescents have received in childhood affection and more consistent disciplinary control from their parents and therefore are better equipped with a framework within which to operate in their struggles of adolescence. In addition, their parents can and do at this time provide a more effective source of security and identification than do the parents of schizophrenics or those with personality disorder.

The evidence here, then, firmly supports the theory that the relationship with the parents, if not *the* most crucial element, is certainly a principal one in the origin and development of these psychiatric illnesses of adolescence. Parents who are sickest, who exhibit the most destructive and numerous pathologic attitudes, have children with the most serious and numerous problems of adolescence and the most severe illnesses. Those who are least sick, with the least pathologic attitudes, have children with less serious illnesses and with far better prognosis for weathering the turmoil of this critical growth period.

SECTION III

THE DIAGNOSTIC DILEMMA

STORIES OF THE DIFFICULTIES in diagnosis in adolescent psychiatry, reaching the proportions of legend, have caused some to urge drastic revision and others to advocate outright abandonment of existing concepts. All admit, however, that some kind of diagnosis, no matter how uncertain, is essential to plan intelligent treatment, since the therapeutic approach to an acute transient illness differs considerably from the approach to a chronic one. Resolution of the dilemma has been impeded to date by the fact that the vacuum existing in psychiatric study of this area has been filled by the psychoanalytic theory that adolescent turmoil causes symptoms to be ubiquitous and transient at this time of life. As a result the psychiatrist, strongly influenced by psychoanalytic theory and having no psychiatric studies to consult, wonders to what extent his patient's clinical picture may be a product of adolescent turmoil and subside and to what extent it may be a manifestation of psychiatric illness and require treatment. Perhaps he falls back upon the diagnosis of adjustment reaction of adolescence, relying too readily on psychoanalytic theory and on the fact that the patient is an adolescent, and not following the clinical evidence far enough. One of the aims of the present study is to redress this imbalance by providing psychiatric data based on the application of existing diagnostic concepts to a group of adolescents, first to crystallize and then to pursue the diagnostic problems and their vicissitudes with the passage of time and later developments.

Section III is addressed to the following questions: How much difficulty is there in determining that a symptomatic adolescent is psychiatrically ill—that is, requires treatment? If he is ill, how much difficulty is there in diagnosis and what are its sources? To

45

what extent are these difficulties resolved as the adolescent moves toward chronological maturity? What bearing do the answers to the foregoing questions have on current theory of the relationship of adolescent turmoil to psychiatric diagnosis?

Let us reiterate, before going further, that we do not consider the diagnostic classification a dogmatic scheme which places the patient in an immutable category. Rather, it is one which, with all its pitfalls and inadequacies, nevertheless tells us useful things about the patient.

When one considers the problems of diagnosis, a few thoughts come to mind that seem to apply regardless of the age of the patient. First, a full-blown classic clinical picture of any of the diagnostic categories is in all likelihood rather easily diagnosed. However, if the patient is in an early stage of illness or his clinical picture is atypical in form, diagnosis becomes harder. Moreover, as discussed in Chapter 2, the definitions of the diagnostic categories themselves create problems. We might expect patients having a typical clinical picture of schizophrenia or character neurosis to present little diagnostic difficulty, while those whose clinical picture is atypical may present the most difficulty. In contrast, patients with personality disorders will probably be the hardest to diagnose regardless of the clinical picture. Ensuing chapters detail the findings by diagnostic category. We will lead off with some general impressions.

The first question is quickly answered: Are these patients in fact psychiatrically ill? With few exceptions there was no doubt that they did not have an adjustment reaction of adolescence but *were* psychiatrically ill and required treatment. The second question, that of diagnostic difficulty, was a different story. Approximately one-half of the patients presented no diagnostic difficulty on the initial interview. This confidence as to diagnosis on the initial interview was later confirmed by the follow-up findings. As might be expected, the degree of diagnostic assurance varied by diagnostic category: we were confident of the diagnosis in 63 per cent of those with character neurosis, 38 per cent of those with schizophrenia and 30 per cent of those with personality disorders.

Thus the character neurosis category showed by far the fewest difficulties in diagnosis, the personality disorder category the most, with the schizophrenic category being in between. Finally, where we did find it hard to make a diagnosis, it was our impression that the difficulties were due as much to the nature of the psychiatric illness itself—i.e., the clarity of the clinical picture and the clarity of the diagnostic category—as to any factor related to adolescent turmoil. It bears repeating that the dilemma was not, as custom suggests, whether the patient had an adjustment reaction of adolescence or a psychiatric illness, but rather, what was the exact diagnosis of his illness?

CHAPTER 5

SCHIZOPHRENIA

> The difficulty in life is the choice.
> The wrong way always seems the more reasonable.
> —George Moore: "The Bending
> of the Bough"

THE DIFFICULTY in the differential diagnosis of schizophrenia lay in the evaluation not of a clinical picture suggestive of adolescent turmoil but rather of one which combined features of a personality disorder and/or a depression with those of schizophrenia. The diagnostic problem was further compounded by the fact that the former could be symptomatic expressions of the latter and that either could exist in an early, more or less amorphous stage. Furthermore, the diagnosis had to be made in an adolescent whose ego structure itself was not fully formed and who, frightened by his impulses, was guarded and uncooperative and often did not reveal enough information for an adequate diagnosis to be made. Small wonder then that in many cases a definitive diagnosis could not be made on the first contact (no matter how intensive) but, as theory implies, had to await changes in the clinical picture that often, but not always, occurred with future developments and the passage of time. In a few cases a definitive diagnosis could not be clearly made even five years later.

Table 3 outlines the initial presenting clinical pictures of the patients for whom schizophrenia was part of the differential diagnosis and also indicates which ones were finally placed in that diagnostic category.

Observing the totals first, we note that schizophrenia, part of the differential diagnosis in twenty-four patients on the initial interview, became the final diagnosis in eighteen. Seven patients (A, Col. 1), or a little less than a third, presented no diagnostic difficulty. Their clinical picture was clearly schizophrenic, with such findings as thinking disorder, ambivalence, autism, and a flat, inappropriate affect. This diagnostic impression on the initial interview was confirmed in all seven by follow-up five years later (Col. 2), when they continued

49

to be clearly diagnosed as schizophrenic. Seventeen, or about two-thirds, presented diagnostic difficulties which revolved about the evaluations of the presenting clinical pictures of personality disorder (eleven patients), depression (five patients), and psychotic adjustment reaction of adolescence (one patient). In Column 2 we observe the outcome or final diagnosis in these patients. Those with the presenting picture of depression as well as the adjustment reaction of adolescence all received a final diagnosis of schizophrenia. Only half of those with a presenting clinical picture of personality disorder were finally diagnosed as schizophrenic (four of the six with a sociopathic presenting picture, and one of the five with a schizoid and passive-aggressive presenting picture). Let us study in more detail the clinical pictures shown in Table 3 to see how they later unraveled. It should be kept in mind that the headings below refer only to initial clinical pictures and not to the final diagnosis.

Table 3. Differential Diagnosis in Schizophrenia

Presenting Symptoms	Col. 1 Initial Clinical Picture (No.)	Col. 2 Final Diagnosis of Schizophrenia (No.)
A. Clear schizophrenic symptomatology	7	7
B. Personality disorder	11	5
1. Sociopath	= 6	= 4
2. Schizoid	= 3	= 1
3. Passive-aggressive	= 2	= 0
C. Depression	5	5
D. Adjustment reaction of adolescence (psychosis)	1	1
Total	24	18

Presenting Clinical Pictures

PERSONALITY DISORDER

The diagnosis of personality disorder will be discussed more fully in a succeeding chapter; here we will describe mainly its differentiation from schizophrenia. As can be seen from Table 3, the eleven patients with a presenting clinical picture of personality disorder were in these subcategories: six sociopathic, three schizoid, and two passive-aggressive. Let us examine each.

Sociopath. Schizophrenia was part of the differential diagnosis in six patients because of the presence of one or more of the following: a history of symptoms in many areas of the personality, and of social difficulty for many years, and findings on examination, such as blunted affect, denial, guardedness and evasiveness, and suspiciousness or inappropriate hostility. None, however, had evidence of inappropriateness of affect or a thinking disorder. In addition, all gave past histories of long duration, one, for example, having had nine years of severe anxiety with conduct disorder in school and at home. The presenting clinical pictures consisted of such manifestations of anxiety as restlessness, concentration difficulty, and insomnia, as well as antisocial behavior, school failure and truancy, and parental conflict.

How were these diagnostic difficulties resolved over the course of time? They were resolved in favor of schizophrenia in two cases, as evidenced by hospitalization for a psychotic breakdown within one year of the initial interview. Here the final diagnosis of schizophrenia was clearly established. They were resolved, but not so clearly, in favor of schizophrenia in two more. On follow-up the first patient did not show the primary features of schizophrenia but was given this diagnosis because of the presence of a flat affect, suspiciousness, a poor social life, pervasive ambivalence and dependency, and sado-masochistic homosexual acting-out. The second patient was hospitalized a year after the initial interview at age sixteen and a half with auditory hallucinations. Review of the hospital record left the diagnosis in doubt between schizophrenia and sociopathic personality with psychosis. The patient improved, was released after a short stay, and when seen at age twenty-one was in prison for having committed a murder. When examined in prison, he was guarded and uncooperative and denied the past history of hallucinations; although his affect was flat, there was no evidence of a thinking disorder. We made a diagnosis of schizophrenia, feeling, however, that it still might possibly be sociopathic personality with a history of psychosis. In the last two patients the difficulties were resolved in favor of sociopathic personality when on follow-up we found a great increase in their antisocial behavior without further development of schizophrenic symptomatology. Nevertheless, in one patient the presence of paranoid elements in the form of suspiciousness and easily roused hostility lent some doubt to the final diagnosis.

The difficulties in diagnosis in these six patients were due to the presence of two elements, sociopathic and schizophrenic, in the clinical picture and not to manifestations of adolescent turmoil. Since sociopaths frequently are isolated and without friends and have blunted affect and psychotic episodes, while schizophrenics often have poor impulse control and acting-out, the combination of the two elements in a guarded, uncooperative adolescent presents the most intricate of riddles to solve. Even on follow-up, the difficulties were clearly resolved in only three cases: two in favor of schizophrenia and one in favor of personality disorder. They were more doubtfully resolved in three: two schizophrenia, one personality disorder. Thus even when the problem is retrospectively reviewed five years later, when the outcome is known, it is hard if not impossible to predict which will take a sociopathic and which a schizophrenic direction. There may, in truth, be no resolution until many years have passed.

The difficulties in diagnosis and prediction, even viewed retrospectively, are illustrated by the following two examples. In both, the initial diagnostic differential was between sociopathic personality with paranoid trends and schizophrenic reaction, but one became schizophrenic and the other sociopathic.

A fifteen-year-old boy gave a history since childhood of conflict with his peers to the point of social isolation, enuresis to age twelve, markedly immature behavior at home characterized by argumentativeness and temper tantrums, irritability, and demanding, attention-getting behavior. Following the death of his mother (when he was eleven), the remarriage of his father (when he was twelve), and a shift to a new school, he became increasingly hostile to his environment and was disturbed besides by emerging sexual impulses. For example, he would slap his face in an effort to prevent erections, feeling that they were unnatural and improper. Whereas previously he had been able to "get by" in school with passing marks, his school performance progressively deteriorated. He became depressed, withdrawing from his few social contacts, and more argumentative and demanding at home. Conflict with peers at school increased, and he was in open conflict with his stepmother. On examination, he was a tall, gangly, immature boy, anxious, tense, depressed, guarded, and evasive but verbalizing considerable resentment against his father and stepmother. His affect was adequate but inappropriate. It was our clinical impression that the differential diagnosis definitely lay between a sociopathic personality with paranoid trends and a paranoid schizophrenic reaction.

Ten months after the initial interview, at the age of sixteen and a half, the patient was placed in a state hospital, at which time he was found to have a flat, inappropriate affect, autistic thinking, and paranoid ideation. He was diagnosed as having a schizophrenic reaction, type undifferentiated. At the age of twenty-one he was still in a state hospital, his illness finally diagnosed as schizophrenia with paranoid and hebephrenic features. Although we had suspected schizophrenia on the initial evaluation, it was not until later that its full-blown development confirmed that diagnosis.

A fifteen-and-a-half-year-old boy, brought to the clinic by his stepmother for truancy and fighting with his peers, gave a history since age twelve, when the father remarried, of gradually increasing truancy, antisocial behavior, and juvenile delinquency. The consultation was precipitated by a worsening of his behavior in the last four months, during which time his stepmother was hospitalized. The patient, developing great hostility to his stepmother and sister, had temper tantrums, threatened to kill them, and pulled a knife on them. At the same time he withdrew from social life and had trouble sleeping, being fearful of attack and occasionally taking a toy gun to bed with him. On examination he was arrogant, boastful, resentful, unkempt, obese, and markedly hostile to and possibly paranoid about his stepmother and sister; in conversation he stressed society's prejudice against the Jewish religion. His mother, a schizophrenic hospitalized since he was six, once had threatened to kill him. The patient had always been a behavioral problem and had difficulty socializing. His early development was slow. He was unable to wash or dress until the age of six, and unable to defend himself against other children. But when he was six, he became an aggressive bully toward his peers and exhibited demanding, attention-getting behavior in school. He was seen in play therapy for a year at the age of ten, where he verbalized little and played mostly with guns. When seen on follow-up at the age of twenty, the patient was living a disorganized life, drifting from job to job, staying out late, "drinking and raising hell," and sleeping during the day. When drinking he had repetitive outbursts of aggressiveness and destructiveness. He suffered recurrent episodes of anxiety, depression, and nightmares of being pursued. He had once held up a bakery to get money to "buy Christmas presents." In addition, the patient had been having a sexual relationship with his aunt for the last three years. On examination, there was no affect or thinking disorder. The final diagnostic impression was sociopathic personality.

Schizoid. Schizophrenia was part of the differential diagnosis in these three patients because of the following: past history of long duration of social withdrawal and lack of assertiveness, and a present-ing clinical picture of concentration difficulty, failures in school, and conflict with the parents although relating to them in a compliant manner. On examination, there was neither inappropriateness of affect nor a thinking disorder. As to later diagnostic developments, only one of these three patients developed a clear-cut schizophrenia; one received a final diagnosis of passive-aggressive personality dis-order and one a final diagnosis of a schizoid personality disorder.

Passive-Aggressive. Schizophrenia was included in the differential diagnosis in these two patients because of blandness of affect, guard-edness, and denial. Further, they had symptoms of depression, pro-crastination, passive-aggressive acting-out in conflict with their parents, concentration difficulty, lack of initiative, and difficulties in managing responsibilities. On closer examination, however, neither inappropri-ateness of affect nor a thinking disorder could be identified. Later follow-up revealed that neither patient developed schizophrenia, both receiving a final diagnosis of a personality disorder, passive-aggressive type.

Unlike those with a sociopathic clinical picture, four out of six of whom became schizophrenic, only one of the five with schizoid or passive-aggressive clinical pictures became schizophrenic. This out-come is quite contrary to our initial impression, which was that the possibility of schizophrenia was more likely in the latter than the former. The combination of social withdrawal, lack of assertiveness, blunted affect, and guardedness and denial makes a strong argument for schizophrenia. According to our findings, the diagnostic caution here should be the reverse of that with the sociopathic picture: al-though the initial evidence for schizophrenia is impressive, the final diagnosis may turn out to be that of a schizoid personality disorder, as is illustrated in the following case history.

A fifteen-year-old, tenth-grade high school student reluctantly came to the clinic under pressure from his mother, who brought him be-cause the school advised a psychiatric evaluation of his deteriorating school performance. In the past two years, since his transfer to an academic high school with high standards, his average had fallen from 85 to 75. He was obsessively concerned about school grades and de-veloped great anxiety when taking tests. Although he had no concen-tration difficulty, he could not retain what he learned.

He was the oldest of three children, the mother preferring his two younger sisters. He did well in school through the sixth grade; however, throughout grade school he was generally unassertive, had trouble socializing, was frequently picked on by his peers, and consequently avoided them. At the beginning of adolescence he grew quite tall and developed feelings of inferiority and awkwardness over his unusual height.

On examination, he appeared preoccupied, withdrawn, and blocked on several occasions; he had a rigid posture, a flat but appropriate affect, some vagueness on abstractions, and no spontaneity. The patient's rigid posture, flatness of affect, lack of spontaneity, blocking, and vagueness of thinking, together with the history of difficulties with assertion and inability to socialize, made us feel rather strongly that the most likely diagnosis was schizophrenia.

When the patient was seen on follow-up at age twenty and a half, he was a senior in business college, seemingly able to function adequately. He still had a hard time learning and experienced anxiety on tests, but these troubles had diminished and his perseverance had increased. He had managed to progress through school, failing an occasional subject each year. His difficulty in socializing remained the same. He spent most of his time alone, rarely going out on dates, and related to his parents in a compliant manner. During examination, he was somewhat guarded in response to questions. He still showed a flat affect, occasional blocking, and a rigid posture when sitting in the chair. There was no evidence at this point of a thinking disorder. Looking at the clinical picture from the vantage point of five years, we felt that the final diagnosis was a schizoid personality disorder and that we had been misled initially by the history of lack of assertion, social difficulty, the rigid posture, and lack of spontaneity.

DEPRESSION

In five patients whose presenting clinical picture was primarily that of depression to the point of suicidal preoccupation or attempt schizophrenia was part of the differential diagnosis because of the presence of a past history of social difficulty and/or findings on examination of blunted affect and guardedness, but again without inappropriate affect or a thinking disorder. Moreover, the past history of a conduct disorder in several suggested the additional possibility that in these patients the depression was only one manifestation of the underlying personality disorder.

On follow-up, three patients, all girls aged seventeen when initially seen, by the time they were twenty had developed a full clinical picture of schizophrenia. In two, seen in treatment over a year, we were unable, despite the most dogged efforts, to make a diagnosis of schizophrenia until the clinical picture itself changed. In a fourth girl depression cleared up in one year with treatment, and on follow-up five years later we felt that the differential diagnosis lay between a schizoid personality disorder and schizophrenia, since she still had a blunted affect and marked vagueness of thinking, but not the fundamental criteria of schizophrenia. In addition, although she functioned adequately, her goals in life were extremely vague. The fifth patient, a boy, demonstrated clear schizophrenic findings in the course of a year's treatment.

On follow-up, therefore, four of the five patients were clearly diagnosed as having schizophrenia and the fifth is probably schizophrenic, although she may have a schizoid personality disorder. The diagnostic difficulty is due to the presence of both depression and schizophrenic features in the clinical picture and not to adolescent turmoil. Depression, long known to be an initial clinical feature of schizophrenia in adolescents, so clouds the presenting clinical picture by its intensity that, standing out like a neon sign in the dark, it obscures the underlying schizophrenic elements and tempts the clinician to settle for a diagnosis of affective disorder. Besides, only when later developments bring the schizophrenic features to the fore is it possible to make the diagnosis. This potent combination, strongly supporting current theory that it takes time to resolve some of these diagnostic problems, warrants both the clinician's respect and his diagnostic caution.

A case example follows.

A seventeen-year-old girl, a high school senior, reported that since the death of her father five years previously she had been obsessively preoccupied with memories of him and had suffered from depression, with suicidal preoccupation. Furthermore, she reported intense hostility toward her mother and eight-year-old brother, nightmares about being killed, headache, and back pains. She had run away from home twice and concomitantly had developed an overly dependent relationship with her male piano teacher. She had a past history of a markedly ambivalent relationship with her overindulgent father and of immature, demanding, and resentful behavior with the rest of the family. Early evidencing musical talent, she had been greatly pressured by her father into a strict regimen of biweekly piano lessons and long hours of practice, so that she had little time for social life and consequently few friends and no satisfaction from her musical training. On examination, she was depressed and tearful; she had blunted affect but no thinking disorder. The differential diagnosis lay between a depression in a personality disorder and schizophrenia, the latter based primarily on her poor social life and the possibility that her preoccupation with thoughts about her father was autistic.

When seen later at the age of twenty, the patient had been graduated from high school, had attended college for one year, and had then run away from home and was living with a man by whom she had had a child. On examination, she was obese, unkempt, depressed, but able to practice the piano and care for her baby. In a few months, however, she became completely disorganized, was overwhelmed with depression punctuated by outbursts of hostility, and, unable to care for her apartment and child, was hospitalized. A year later, when pregnant for the second time, she again became disorganized and was again admitted to the hospital, where she had dreams of murdering her baby and much difficulty in controlling her conscious hostile impulses toward the child. She was finally diagnosed as having schizophrenia, paranoid type.

Again, the schizophrenic elements in this patient were present on the initial interview, but they either were masked by the depression or actually at that time were only a minor theme and it took later developments to bring them to the fore.

ADJUSTMENT REACTION OF ADOLESCENCE

There was a singular exception among the entire group of seventy-two, in that the differential diagnosis included the category of adjustment reaction of adolescence. His case story follows.

The patient, a sixteen-year-old boy, at age twelve had become anxious, done poorly in school, and withdrawn from social contacts. At sixteen he suddenly developed, to a delusional degree, a common preoccupation of adolescents: that people thought circles under his eyes indicated masturbation. On examination, he was guarded and evasive and had a blunted but appropriate affect and no thinking disorder. The differential diagnostic impression lay between adjustment reaction of adolescence (psychotic) and a schizophrenic reaction, probably paranoid type.

Follow-up at age twenty-one raised some question about the diagnosis. Without treatment his delusion had disappeared and his concentration difficulty improved enough for him to graduate from high school. Under severe conflict with an alcoholic mother, he had left home and was living alone. He had developed an interest in electronics and religion. Though he had dated, he had recently broken up with a girl friend and otherwise his social life was minimal. On examination, he showed vagueness of thinking, guardedness, and blunted affect and possible paranoid trends. Our final impression was that the diagnosis was schizophrenia which had compensated at a level permitting the patient to function.

The Diagnostic Dilemma

Let us return now to the subject to which this chapter was addressed. We did have considerable trouble making the diagnosis of schizophrenia. In only about one-third of the patients was the diagnosis clearly evident on initial interview. In the other two-thirds, the diagnostic difficulties were due, not to adolescent turmoil, but to the fact that the presenting clinical pictures contained features of schizophrenia combined with features of either a personality disorder or a depression. The dilemma is compounded by the fact that the latter may be symptomatic expressions of the former, either may exist in an early unformed stage, and the diagnosis must be made in an adolescent whose ego structure is in a state of flux and who, frightened by his impulses, is guarded and uncooperative and often does not reveal information adequate for a firm diagnosis.

In many of these cases, moreover, the final diagnosis can be made only when later developments have clarified the clinical picture, and in some the diagnosis continues unresolved. In the personality disorder group, if the presenting clinical picture was sociopathic rather than schizoid or passive-aggressive, it was more likely to turn out to be schizophrenia, since three of the six in the former category became clearly schizophrenic, while only one of the five patients in the two latter categories did so. On the other hand, the presence of social difficulty, lack of assertiveness, blunted affect, guardedness, and denial in those with a clinical picture of a schizoid or passive-aggressive disorder may not lead to a schizophrenic diagnosis. The findings in these patients give very little comfort to the clinician, for they are the most difficult to diagnose. When his patient's clinical picture contains the elements of both schizophrenia and depression or personality disorder, after pursuing his diagnostic labor to the utmost, he must rest content for the moment and live with the ambiguity regarding diagnosis but remain alert to future developments that will resolve his dilemma.

CHAPTER 6

PERSONALITY DISORDERS

For on the one hand lay Scylla, and on the other
mighty Charybdis in terrible wise sucked down the
salt sea water.
As often as she belched it forth, like a cauldron on
a great fire she would seethe up through all her
troubled deeps, and overhead the spray fell on the
tops of either cliff.

—Homer: *The Odyssey,*
Book XII

THE DIAGNOSIS of a personality disorder involves a journey as
arduous and treacherous as that of Ulysses, complete with its own
Scylla and Charybdis. These treacheries, some unique to growth and
development in adolescence and others unique to the psychopathology
of personality disorders, further complicate the making of a diagnosis that is difficult enough to do at any time in life. This chapter
defines the term *personality disorder* and describes the obstacles to
diagnosis created both by its psychopathology and by the developmental character of adolescence. Chapter 7 presents the prominent
themes involved in clinical differential diagnosis, and Chapter 8 applies these themes to the subtypes of personality disorder.

The concept of personality disorders used was that described in the
American Psychiatric Association manual: disorders characterized by
developmental defects or pathologic trends in the structure of the
personality which are manifested by a lifelong pattern of action or
behavior, rather than by mental or emotional symptoms [2]. The personality disorders are descriptively subdivided, partly on the basis of
the dynamics of personality development, into three subgroups: personality pattern disturbances, personality trait disturbances, and sociopathic personality. Patients in the first group have had deep-seated
disturbances with little room for regression without development of a
psychosis. Those in the second and third groups may lose their emotional equilibrium and independence under stress and regress to a lower
level of adjustment, but they still may function without developing a
psychosis.

Table 4 presents the APA manual's [2] outline of the various sub-types of personality disorder.

Table 4. Subtypes of Personality Disorder*

Personality Pattern Disturbances	Personality Trait Disturbances	Sociopathic Personality
1. Inadequate personality	1. Emotionally unstable personality	1. Antisocial
2. Schizoid personality	2. Passive-aggressive personality A. Passive-dependent B. Passive-aggressive C. Aggressive	2. Dissocial
3. Cyclothymic personality	3. Compulsive personality	3. Sexual deviation
4. Paranoid personality	4. Personality trait disturbances—other	4. Addiction

* From the American Psychiatric Association, *Diagnostic and Statistical Manual of Mental Disorders*, 1962 [2].

The first difficulties in diagnosis we encountered, described below, related on the one hand to the psychopathology of the personality disorder and on the other hand to the developmental character of adolescence.

Psychopathology of Personality Disorder

The term *personality disorder* embraces less homogeneity than applies to the schizophrenias or the psychoneuroses, and has tended to become a psychiatric wastebasket. Though personality disorders share a common etiology—a developmental defect in ego structure—the clinical manifestations on which the diagnosis must be made vary from schizoid or paranoid behavior to emotionally inadequate or antisocial behavior. The APA manual by definition clearly separates these disorders, but in actual clinical practice differentiation becomes difficult because patients often have manifestations of several disorder categories and the borderlines between categories are indistinct. The key word is *admixtures*. Moreover, the diagnosis is based on patterns of behavior rather than emotional or mental symptoms. In schizophrenia, for example, not only are disturbing symptoms such as delusions and hallucinations frequently reported but there are also objective, observable findings on examination, such as a thinking disorder, autism, and a flat, inappropriate affect. Similarly, in the character neuroses the patient's anxiety, depression, and/or phobia causing him great distress are definitely reported. Since these symptoms can often be observed during the interview, a prompt and uncomplicated diagnosis is possible. In contrast, in the personality disorder, although the patient's behavior patterns can, to a certain extent, be observed in the interview, careful history taking is likely to be required in order to delineate such patterns of behavior as paranoid sensitivity, passive-aggressiveness, or egocentricity. Therefore, the diagnosis depends less on the observations of the skilled person in the interview than on the history obtained from psychiatrically unskilled people—family friends, social workers, teachers, and school records.

The diagnostic problem is further compounded by the fact that, the psychopathology militates against obtaining a good history in a disorder that must be diagnosed largely by history. Contrary to the description in the APA manual, most of our patients did suffer often from both anxiety and other distress which, probably because of their low tolerance for such discomfort, they would report quite freely and which could be readily observed in the interview. However, they did *not* report, perhaps because of denial or unawareness, the patterns of behavior essential to the diagnosis, such as passive-aggressiveness and schizoid or sociopathic behavior. In other words, the patient was least likely to report the very aspects of his reactions and behavior necessary to the diagnosis. Consequently, not only the report of the present illness but also the patient's own description of his symptoms in the past contained many distortions, contradictions, denials, and omissions.

Interviews with the mother produced similar inadequacies in the history, apparently owing to two factors: the type of behavior exhibited by the patient and the degree of awareness of the mother. In the recognition of passive-dependency, for instance, it takes a perceptive and knowledgeable observer to notice that the degree of dependency expected in childhood is not lessening as it normally should with age. Yet frequently not until late adolescence, seventeen and older, does this feature become obvious to the mother. There seems to be a spectrum of awareness spreading from antisocial behavior, of which the mothers are most aware, through passive-aggressive behavior to passive-dependent behavior, of which they are least aware. This lack of awareness may be due to a number of factors: The mother, often having schizophrenia or a personality disorder herself, may be completely uninterested in or actually unconsciously promoting the patient's behavior. Moreover, many guilt-laden mothers may deny the presence of these patterns as a problem. Others may be so unconcerned with or rejecting of the patient, that they are not attuned to the significance of his behavior. Lastly, a number will be blinded to admitting to a child's behavior from which they are deriving unconscious gratification.

These formidable obstacles to diagnosis—all related to the psychopathology of the personality disorders, the heterogeneity of the category, the reliance on history where it is difficult to obtain—are possibly more important factors than adolescent turmoil in the widespread diagnostic confusion. However, let us now try to set apart certain obstacles to diagnosis related to the developmental character of adolescence.

Developmental Character of Adolescence

The recognition of a personality disorder is easier in an adult than in an adolescent because the discrepancy between adult status and infantile behavior may be quite clearly discerned. The line is blurred in adolescence, where personality development is not yet complete and a certain amount of immature behavior must be expected; the dependency need, too, only gradually decreases and rarely in smooth gradations from early adolescence to emancipation. Thus it is hard to evaluate dependency as a pathologic trend important to the diagnosis of personality disorder unless it is prominent. Actually, a certain degree of dependency is a natural phenomenon of adolescence.

The developmental character of adolescence poses another problem: the diagnosis of a defect in development must be made before the developmental process is finished. Theoretically, since the process is not complete, later developments might drastically alter the picture.

However, since the defect in ego development essential to the diagnosis occurs in the early stages of development, during the first few years of life, and forms the basic framework for later adolescent changes, it is highly unlikely that the latter will essentially alter the fundamental defect. This hypothesis is borne out by our finding that in most patients the defect in development began very early in life and persisted up to and through adolescence.

General Diagnostic Considerations

Before turning to the details of the clinical review, let us consider for a moment the entire group of forty-three patients with a final diagnosis of personality disorder. We excluded two from this review, feeling that their past historys did not compare in adequacy with those of the others, leaving a total of forty-one upon whom to base the findings. In twelve of the forty-one, or about 30 per cent, we were confident on the initial interview that their diagnosis was a personality disorder, though in only three (two sociopaths, one passive-dependent) could we be fairly sure of the exact subtype. In twenty-nine, or 70 per cent, we had some doubt on the initial interview as to whether the diagnosis was personality disorder. The difficulties in establishing this diagnosis are further indicated by the fact that on final clinical review five years later, although we felt confident on the final diagnosis in twenty-eight, there still were thirteen, or roughly one-third, about whom we still had some uncertainty, mostly as to the exact subtype of personality disorder.

To summarize then: We are attempting to identify a developmental defect in a patient who is himself in a stage of development. The identification is based on patterns of behavior rather than observable symptoms, in a patient who presents dramatic complaints of distress but denies or is unaware of his behavioral patterns, with a mother who may be unconsciously encouraging and also unaware of these patterns for any number of reasons. It bears repeating that the diagnostic difficulties are due as much to the psychopathology of the personality disorders as to adolescent turmoil.

The clinician's only safeguard in this web of complications is his realization of the problem and his willingness to pursue a developmental history until he has detected and uncovered the whole story. An important by-product of this study has been our heightened awareness of the difficulties involved in making the diagnosis of personality disorder and therefore our increased alertness and persistence in gathering the necessary evidence, which has notably increased our efficiency in spotting pathologic behavior patterns, whatever the "treachery" of their admixtures with the growth and developmental stages of adolescence.

The above discussion raises the question as to how much adolescence, as a phase of development, has been bearing the onus for diagnostic difficulties which are due less to adolescence and more to the problems inherent in the psychopathology of personality disorder. This question is particularly relevant when one considers that most adolescents seen by psychiatrists, either in clinics or in private practice, probably have personality disorders.

CHAPTER 7

DIFFERENTIAL DIAGNOSIS OF PERSONALITY DISORDERS

> So she led me in and set me on a chair with studs
> of silver, a goodly carven chair, and beneath was a
> footstool for the feet. And she made me a potion in
> a golden cup, that I might drink, and she also put
> a charm therein, in the evil counsel of her heart.
> —Homer: *The Odyssey,*
> Book X

HAVING MANAGED, like Ulysses, to avoid Scylla and to circumvent Charybdis, and therefore having obtained the necessary clinical evidence for a diagnosis, we now move on to the next obstacle, akin to Circe—the difficulties in differential diagnosis once the evidence has been collected. These differential difficulties arose at two levels in our study. First, when the diagnosis of personality disorder itself was definite in twelve cases, decision as to the specific subtype was difficult in nine of these, the choice usually lying between a passive-aggressive and one of the other subtypes, most often the sociopathic (six cases). Second, when the diagnosis of personality disorder was in doubt (twenty-nine cases) we had trouble differentiating the disorder from a character neurosis (eighteen cases), from a schizophrenia (six cases), and from epilepsy (five cases). Thus, by far the major theme of diagnostic difficulty (43 per cent, or eighteen cases) is the differentiation of a personality disorder from a character neurosis. Closer study of this problem revealed that it could be more exactly stated as follows: The difficulties are in perceiving the personality disorder that underlies and is masked by a dramatic façade of psychoneurotic symptoms. Incidentally, Beck [8] reports this decision to be equally troublesome in adults.

As if the foregoing complications were not sufficient, there is one more—the influence of a severely pathologic parent (usually the mother) on the presenting clinical picture. If an adolescent with mild features of personality disorder develops symptoms in conflict with an obviously pathologic parent, the temptation is to undervalue the importance of the features of personality disorder and ascribe the patient's problem to conflict with the parent. This possibility was not borne out in our cases: almost without exception, we found that the most determinative element in the diagnosis was neither the conflict with the parent, nor the presenting symptomatology, but the underlying personality disorder.

Since we have already discussed the differentiation of a personality disorder from schizophrenia (Chapter 5), we will only briefly refer to it again. The diagnostic problems presented by epilepsy will be presented in Chapter 10. This chapter focuses on three difficulties: differentiating a specific subtype, diagnosing the underlying personality disorder beneath the psychoneurotic symptoms, and assessing the influence of the pathologic parent in the presenting clinical picture.

Determining the Subtype

The difficulties involved in differentiating a specific subtype were due to the presence of manifestations of more than one subtype without sufficient evidence to distinguish one from the other or to decide which was predominant. Furthermore, the subtype which seemed minor on the initial interview might be in an early stage of development and come to full flower later. For example, a patient's predominant manifestations on initial interview might be passive-aggressiveness with some mild antisocial behavior, and as he got older the antisocial aspect of his disorder would come to the fore. Or there might be no evidence of a sociopathic disorder, which would nevertheless make its appearance later; or the converse could happen: flagrant sociopathic behavior would subside and passive-aggressive behavior come to the fore. In these nine cases, the main difficulty (in six) was to differentiate a passive-aggressive subtype from either a sociopathic type or an inadequate personality. In the remaining three, the problem was to differentiate a passive-aggressive disorder from a schizoid disorder in one case and from a paranoid disorder in another, and in the final case to differentiate a hysterical character disorder from a sociopathic disorder.

As a baseline for comparison we describe first a case that offered no diagnostic difficulty.

A sixteen-year-old boy, in a setting of marked conflict with his mother and father, gave a history since childhood of procrastination, lying, lack of responsibility, difficulty in controlling impulses, nail-biting and thumb-sucking. At age thirteen and a half, when the family moved to a poor neighborhood and his mother increased her pressure on him, he became depressed, engaged in truancy, failed all his subjects at school, and was referred because he had not been in school for thirty days. Though he feared he would get into delinquent activities, he had actually been stealing for the last three years, with the move to the poor neighborhood. The mother, who had always been oversolicitous as well as restrictive, carefully checking on the patient's study habits, clothing, and how he spent his free time, became even more so and increased her pressure. The patient responded with depression and resentment, reporting constant arguments with his mother (and subsequent punishment) and also resentment at his father's siding with his mother. For example, he stated: "She nags me about everything; if I put on the wrong shirt she disapproves and we fight. She gets on my nerves; she curses me. I think I am cracking up." On examination there was further evidence of depression and tension, but his affect was normal and there was no thinking disorder.

The patient continued to have almost daily altercations with his mother and was more and more frequently a truant from school. Eventually he dropped out and enlisted in the army at the age of eighteen. Here he was soon in serious trouble. He was court-martialed and received a suspended sentence, and was finally discharged for behavioral problems, at the age of twenty.

Since that time he has had chronic difficulty at work, being able to hold a job for a short time only. The conflict he had with his mother is now present as a smoldering and too readily expressed resentment, and he is suspicious toward any figure of authority. At the age of twenty, one year prior to the final interview, he married. It seemed clear that he transferred his dependency needs from his mother to his wife, who, however, has almost left him on several occasions because of his temper outbursts. He remains impulsive, has not learned to control his fierce temper, and is irresponsible and extravagant in handling money. In addition, he suffers from anxiety, depression, nail-biting, and tension headaches.

In the next case, the diagnosis of personality disorder was definite, but the subtype was unclear.

A fifteen-and-a-half year-old boy, a high school junior, complained that learning was being crammed down his throat by his teachers, whom he openly defied and talked back to. He disliked his peers and had been truant from school for two months. He recounted a similar episode of misbehavior at age twelve and a half, when he had dropped out of school for four months but returned after a period of psychiatric treatment. Much of his truancy was a frank rebellion against his parents, whose every effort or lack of effort in his behalf roused his anger and disdain. He complained of insomnia, anorexia, and episodes of depression. He had always attended school unwillingly and had recurrent gastrointestinal disorders. His behavior throughout childhood was characterized by irresponsibility, self-centeredness, and temper tantrums. He also had suffered ear and mastoid infections intermittently since the age of three. Despite this turbulent history of physical and emotional problems, he managed to attend school frequently enough to progress from grade to grade and at the same time to maintain a fairly active social life.

On examination, he was egocentric, arrogant, belligerent, anxious, and depressed and bit his fingernails, but he had no affect or thinking disorder. Our impression at the time was that the history of self-centeredness, the irresponsibility with temper tantrums since early childhood, and the acting-out of rebellion through truancy in adolescence, together with the findings on examination, strongly supported the diagnosis of a personality disorder, though the specific subtype was uncertain and lay between a passive-aggressive, aggressive, and a sociopathic disorder.

When seen on first follow-up, at the age of seventeen and a half, he had been graduated from high school and had attended a local college for half a term but had dropped out, being unable to sit in classes because of restlessness and unable to do the homework because of procrastination. Four months prior to the interview he had taken a job as a clerk in a stock brokerage company. He had trouble going to work and had had absences for as long as a week. He was taking a course in financing but experiencing the same inability to do his homework. He continued to have disagreements and quarrels with his mother, with his peers, and with girls. He reported that he was anxious and impulsive, and aware of being self-centered and inconsiderate; his nail-biting, insomnia, moodiness, depression, and lying persisted.

When seen for the second follow-up, at age twenty, he had worked for several years and had recently resumed college as a freshman at the urging of the girl to whom he had recently become engaged. Though he had done well in summer school the previous year, at the time of the interview he found the pace too slow, was bored, and planned to drop out. He remained resentful toward and in conflict with his parents, and with all authority figures. During his recurrent depressive episodes, which could last from a week to a month, he felt numb, tired, and lazy. He said he required a great deal of sleep, but he would sleep from seven to eight-thirty in the evening and then read until two or three in the morning. He had great trouble in getting out of bed in the morning, was irritable and tense, smoked two packs of cigarettes a day, remained impulsive, moody, had headaches, complained of loneliness, and showed some compulsive trends. On examination, he was guarded, hostile, and defiant.

The final diagnosis was a sociopathic personality disorder, based on his narcissism, impulsiveness and acting-out, low frustration tolerance, chronic conflicts with authority that resulted in chronic work difficulties, and shallow relationship with people.

These two cases suggest that, in some sociopathic personality disorders, it is possible to have a fairly firm confidence about the diagnosis on the initial interview. That this may not always be the actual situation is indicated by the following case.

The patient, a fifteen-year-old boy who was a freshman in high school, had returned home from boarding school and entered public school for the first time. Since childhood he had been in marked conflict with his nagging mother, whom he passively resisted. At school he was failing French and mathematics. There was a history of behavioral difficulty since age eight, manifested by poor conduct and failing work at school. He was switched from school to school, had one year of psychotherapy at age nine, and at age ten, at camp, was reported to have engaged in homosexual play. At age twelve to fourteen, when at boarding school, he gave a history of homosexual activity and of being the leader of a group involved in stealing. When he was eleven and a half, his father had separated from and divorced his mother, and since then his conflict with his mother had worsened.

On examination, he was evasive and denied having problems. His affect was somewhat blunted, but he showed no thinking disorder. Our initial impression, based on the history of poor conduct, homosexual play, and stealing since age ten, was between a sexual perversion—homosexuality—and a personality disorder, possibly sociopathic in type. At this point we would have predicted that this patient could go either way—but certainly not what eventually did happen.

When seen on first follow-up at age eighteen, the patient reported that his behavior had changed remarkably. He had spent his fifteenth summer with his father in South America and the next summer with his uncle on a ranch, with both of whom he got along well. At school he had done borderline work, failing subjects he was not interested in but then making up the work and managing to pass. He had developed migraine headaches, but at age seventeen "the era of bad feeling with his mother subsided," and he stopped "pulling stunts" since he was "now a man." He was intent on pursuing a career in commercial art, was trying to work harder at school, felt more concerned and guilty about his behavior with his mother, and currently had a job in a supermarket. He was active socially; however, he never dated girls and felt that his peers were too preoccupied with sexual matters. He felt close to and extremely affectionate toward his father and was more considerate of his mother, feeling that though she was oversolicitous she was more relaxed with him.

On second follow-up, at the age of twenty, the patient was enrolled in an art school and was then living away from home. He had been graduated from high school at age eighteen but, not having enough credits for college, had gone to night school for a year and a half to make up this deficit. He wanted to be an artist like his father and worked well as an artist's assistant during the summer. For the past six months he had had insomnia and occasional nightmares. He still had little interest in girls, dating very infrequently, had not had sexual intercourse, but claimed to masturbate freely without guilt feelings. On examination, he was somewhat anxious, had a poor memory for and indeed denied his past difficulties, but showed no affect or thinking disorder. His acting-out had disappeared.

Our final diagnosis was personality disorder, type undetermined. Though some evidence suggests the possibility of an underlying homosexuality, there was not enough to confirm this diagnosis. Further follow-up would be necessary to identify the specific subtype of his personality disorder.

This case is instructive in both the presenting clinical picture and in its outcome. The former is quite similar to that of the two previous cases; all three had a past history of a long duration of conduct disorders, some antisocial behavior, and acting-out of conflict with parents. On this basis, one might have predicted a sociopathic development, but the outcome was otherwise. On reviewing the case again to find an explanation for this unexpected turn of events we found several possible factors: (1) the presence of the father in the home until the patient was eleven and a half years old; (2) an extraordinarily good relationship with the father and obvious identification with him; (3) the opportunity to spend time with his father and the father's returning home; (4) many sublimations shown even on the initial interview, i.e., interest in art, stamps, coins, model cars, airplanes, painting and drawing—in other words, an already considerable ego development; (5) the mother's multiple illnesses and her personality, which involved a great deal of oversolicitousness and nagging about school. Suffice it to say at this point that in many instances the clinician should rest content with a definite diagnosis of personality disorder only, letting the subtype await future developments.

Discerning a Personality Disorder Behind Psychoneurotic Symptoms

The next diagnostic difficulty, the differentiation from a character neurosis, was due to the presence of manifestations of both a psychoneurosis or a character neurosis and a personality disorder. There were several variations on this theme: Manifestations of both could appear in the present illness and in past history, or only one would appear in the past history, or only one might appear in the present illness with manifestations of both apparent in the past history. Psychoneurotic symptoms, whenever they occurred in the past, went through a period of remission and then exacerbation during the present illness, giving the latter a heavy psychoneurotic coloring which tempted the clinician, especially if the manifestations of personality disorder were mild in both present illness and past history, into disregarding the underlying personality disorder and therefore not pursuing the developmental history adequately enough to establish the diagnosis.

The first case contains manifestations of both psychoneurosis and personality disorder in the present illness and the past history.

One year prior to admission the patient, a fourteen-and-a-half-year-old boy, a freshman at a public high school, had a recurrence of spells of anxiety associated with vomiting and social withdrawal to the extent that he began to truant, his schoolwork deteriorated, and he was required to repeat a year. He was then transferred from a Catholic to a public school, apparently to no avail. The father died when the patient was a year old, and he is the oldest of three children. When he was five his mother remarried, at which time he developed enuresis that persisted until age ten. When this subsided he began to have anxiety and vomiting spells associated with social withdrawal whenever under stress. The mother, oversolicitous and overindulgent, once took him out of his Boy Scout troop because she was afraid something would happen to him on hikes. His stepfather, contrary to the mother, is quite rigid and strict. The patient fought with both his sister and half brother. During his childhood the patient always attended parochial schools, where he did borderline work, and, though never active socially, he had a number of outside interests, including swimming, playing ball, and horseback riding. Up to three weeks prior to admission he shared a room with his sister.

On examination, he was found to be markedly immature, evasive, anxious and tense, and suffering from concentration difficulty. There were hints which could not be developed about possible sexual problems relating to masturbation. The prominent past and present history of psychoneurotic symptoms, the obvious anxiety and tension and the vomiting spells, and the mild personality disorder manifestations—enuresis, social withdrawal, and truancy in the present illness—suggested a psychoneurotic reaction.

Follow-up interviews with the mother only, since the patient was unwilling to come, revealed progressive development of a sociopathic disorder. At age seventeen the patient had left high school, enlisted in the Air Force, and then been discharged as unfit for service (in the Air Force he had received a sentence for falling asleep while on guard duty.) He attended mechanics school, where he began to cut classes, and was indecisive and unable to settle on school or work. He came into greater conflict with his stepfather and spent most of his time out of the house. His anxiety, tension, and vomiting, however, disappeared.

When he was twenty-two, the mother reported that he was unable to continue in school, had sporadic employment, led an aimless life, had a police record with charges against him for drag racing, speeding, stealing hubcaps (he had stolen fifty hubcaps with two other boys), and leaving the scene of an accident. He had twenty-five convictions for driving without a license and had served a twenty-five-day sentence. At home he was withdrawn from both parents and in marked conflict with his stepfather. He seemed to exhibit little anxiety over his difficulties with the law. When hauled before the court, he made no attempt to defend himself. He was driving an uninsured and unregistered car without a license.

Although personality disorder elements were noted on the initial interview, these were so far overshadowed by the psychoneurotic symptoms that our initial impression was determined by the latter. As later events demonstrated, the former elements were the more fundamental. The final diagnosis is probably sociopathic personality.

In contrast to the two cases already described, possibly this patient did not actually develop his sociopathic personality disorder until later, so that it would have been impossible on the initial interview to predict the outcome.

The next patient had intense psychoneurotic symptoms only in the present illness, but a past history of manifestations of personality disorder, which were, however, of mild intensity, along with some psychophysiologic symptoms.

The patient was a fourteen-and-a-half-year-old girl, who six months prior to admission had had an acute onset of anxiety and vomiting after failing her Regents Examinations. This had occurred in the setting of the marriage of a brother to whom she was closely attached, and of a classmate's kidding her about pregnancy. These episodes were followed several weeks prior to admission by anxiety, particularly intense in crowds and in the classroom, and accompanied by polyuria and urgency of such a degree that she had to leave abruptly to go to the bathroom. On one such occasion, when a boy blocked her exit she attacked him. She then briefly disappeared from home, following which the intensity of her anxiety required her to be hospitalized for four weeks. She was discharged with the diagnosis of a conversion reaction.

When first seen by us, she appeared immature, anxious, and hypermotile but had a blunted and somewhat inappropriate affect, much denial, and depression. The past history was negative except for dysmenorrhea with menarche at the age of ten, during which time she also experienced some anxiety at school. Interviews revealed the girl's mother to be immature, with many phobias, prudish about sexual matters, socially isolated, and separated from her husband since the patient was a year and a half old. She had overindulged the patient, expecting a great deal of her, and had frequent outbursts of hostility because of the daughter's inability to meet these expectations. On initial evaluation of the patient her own dramatic phobic symptoms—learned in part, no doubt, from her mother—so clouded the underlying dependency and passivity that we were misled into an impression of a psychoneurotic reaction with phobic and hysterical features.

After the initial evaluation the patient did not return to school. She received home instruction for two years, and at age sixteen and a half, when she was four months pregnant, she married a Puerto Rican boy. Her phobic symptoms diminished, perhaps because she lived a markedly restricted life. Her husband appeared to be immature and overdependent on his parental family. There was great conflict in the marriage, the patient and her husband having physical fights. In the setting of increasing frequency of these fights, the patient became depressed and made one suicidal attempt.

By the time of the second follow-up, the patient had had another child, at age nineteen. She experienced no difficulty in caring for her children, though she remained dependent on her mother, who assisted her. She had almost no social life and few outside interests, and was also excessively dependent on her husband. She complained of anxiety, headaches, and depression and described her "acting-out" when depressed or angry. She was thinking of returning to work in a factory where she had been for a short period of time before she was married.

The passage of time, which saw a subsidence of the dramatic phobic symptoms, helped expose and clearly outline that part of the patient's problem that had been obscured, i.e., the underlying personality disorder, passive-dependent type. In retrospect, we feel that a more diligent search for this in the initial interview might have led to the proper diagnosis.

The last case illustrates manifestations of mild personality disorder both in the present illness and in the past history.

An eighteen-and-a-half-year-old boy, a high school senior, had hemophilia which had required four hospitalizations in the last two years. In the last three years, under the pressure of being a pawn in conflict between mother and father, he developed anxiety, tension, irritability, episodic depression, suicidal thoughts, and thought of running away. His lifelong difficulties in assuming the initiative became worse, and he had failed two subjects in school in the previous term. He later reported that several homosexual experiences had occurred at this time. We were severely handicapped in our evaluation of this case on the initial interview by not being able to interview the mother. However, we did see her on the first follow-up interview, when she described such manifestations of personality disorder in her son from early childhood as mild conduct disorder in school, temper tantrums during which he would hurt himself if he didn't get his own way, and some occasional minor stealing in early adolescence. He had always been self-centered, arrogant, demanding, and overdependent on his mother.

On examination, the predominant impression was of depression with some anxiety and passivity. In addition, he had some effeminate mannerisms. There was no affect or thinking disorder. The prominence of the depression together with the precipitating factors derived from the conflict between the parents and the long-standing physical illness again led us to underestimate the role of the underlying personality disorder in favor of a tentative diagnosis of psychoneurosis, mixed with anxiety and depression.

When seen five years later, at age twenty-three, the patient recently graduated from a school of design, was looking for a job and had been married for eighteen months. Though he had received a "B" average in school, he had great difficulty in being prompt and suffered from procrastination, rarely finishing his work until the last moment and then in a great flurry of tension. He described his relationship with his wife as good, though she dominated him and complained that he did not show her enough affection. The patient was resentful toward both his mother and his father and constantly irritated by his wife's parents also. He reported anxiety and depression with periods of hopelessness, tension, insomnia, and restlessness, as well as his need to be dominated and directed. He voiced resentment at "having to do everything himself" and experienced marked feelings of inadequacy about being an architect, a father, and a husband. Again the passage of time had disclosed the patient's personality disorder, passive-aggressive type, in his dependency, passivity, lack of initiative, and need to be directed and dominated by his wife.

The presence of physical disease (hemophilia), the precipitating factors, of conflict between the parents, and the dramatic presenting symptoms of anxiety and depression, combined with the mild personality disorder manifestations in the past, all tended to mislead us in the direction of a diagnosis of psychoneurosis rather than to identify the underlying personality disorder.

The Problems with Schizophrenia

The third diagnostic difficulty (six cases), was in deciding between a personality disorder and schizophrenia. This manifested itself in two ways. First, in three patients, in whom symptomatology was present in many areas of the personality without the primary features of schizophrenia, the diagnosis was between a sociopathic personality and schizophrenia. Second, in three patients, who had symptoms of a schizoid personality disorder without the fundamental features of schizophrenia, the diagnosis was between schizophrenia and a schizoid personality disorder. For a fuller discussion we refer the reader to Chapter 5.

Effect of a Pathologic Parent

We come now to the last diagnostic difficulty: evaluating the influence on the presenting clinical picture of conflict with a pathologic parent. This factor, just like psychoneurotic symptoms, tended to seduce the clinician away from a diagnosis of personality disorder and toward attributing the patient's problems to the obvious conflict with the pathologic parent. We found, however, that the patient's problem was not an acute one related to conflict with his parent, but rather a long-standing one related to defects in personality development. This suggests that the more fundamental influence of the pathologic parent on the clinical picture lies not in the current conflict but in the detrimental effect early in life on the development of the patient's ego structure. Without question, this preexistent situation can be aggravated in the present by any number of factors, one of them being the onset of adolescence. The following case illustrates the difficulty that conflict with the pathologic mother can impose on the evalution of the presenting clinical picture.

A fifteen-year-old boy, a high school junior, had come into increasing discord and disagreement with his mother and sister since age eleven following his development of kyphosis scoliosis, which restricted his physical activity. He became withdrawn, rebellious, antagonistic, and resentful. In the heat of an altercation, his domineering, oversolicitous, pressuring mother would occasionally hit him and he would strike back. On one occasion he ran away from home. His school marks had deteriorated from excellent to barely passing. He had a history of a congenital clubfoot which required a cast from age six weeks to fourteen months, and alopecia at age eleven. His father had died when the boy was two years old.

On examination, the patient was anxious, tense, vague, guarded, and evasive, particularly about the conflict with his mother, and showed an inability to concentrate. The absence of a past history of manifestations of personality disorder, together with the violent quality of the conflict with the pathologic mother, suggested that the patient was reacting to this conflict by rebellion with resultant acting-out and anxiety. On follow-up, however, we found that when he left home the rebellion disappeared but his anxiety and school difficulties persisted and seemed at this point to be related to an underlying lack of ambition and drive, inability to study, procrastination, and daydreaming.

When seen at age twenty, he had been graduated from high school and was repeating his junior year of college. He again complained of difficulty in concentration, distractibility, restlessness, daydreaming, procrastination, general "nervousness," excessive smoking, occasional body tics, and anxiety over sexual conflicts. He had never had intercourse and had had a premature ejaculation when once he tried. He also felt inadequate with his male friends. As the dramatic impact of the conflict with the mother subsided, the more basic aspects of the personality disorder came to the fore.

To summarize: This tangled net of obstacles to the diagnosis of a personality disorder in adolescents can best be appreciated by noting that at times the clinician may have to pick his way through all of them combined in one case—psychoneurotic symptoms, schizophrenic symptoms, personality disorder symptoms, epilepsy, and conflict with a pathologic mother. He must keep himself alert in order to avoid pressing the developmental history into the wrong mold. And in some cases only the passage of time will resolve the often more than two-horned dilemma.

CHAPTER 8

SUBTYPES OF PERSONALITY DISORDERS

> Thither we sailed, and some God guided us through
> the night, for it was dark and there was no light to
> see, a mist lying deep about the ships, nor did the
> moon show her light from heaven, but was shut in
> with clouds.
>
> —Homer: *The Odyssey*,
> Book IX

CHAPTERS 6 and 7, viewing the personality disorders as a single diagnostic entity, described the obstacles to diagnosis relating to difficulties in obtaining the evidence, as well as the difficulties in differential diagnosis once the evidence has been obtained. Since the personality disorders are a loosely defined entity made up of heterogeneous subtypes, this chapter, reporting our findings by subtype, discusses the diagnostic difficulties encountered and whether they were resolved with time. It poses the following questions: Looking at a five-year history of a group with sociopathic personality or a passive-aggressive personality disorder, what can we discern as the differential possibilities on the initial interview? What happened to these with the passage of time? The chapter then concludes our consideration of personality disorders by describing the patients who continued to show residual diagnostic difficulties even five years later.

Table 5 presents the final diagnosis of personality disorder by specific subtype for thirty-six patients. We have again excluded the five patients with epilepsy, who will be considered in Chapter 10.

We observe that the passive-aggressive subtype is by far the most common, constituting more than half the total group; the sociopathic subtype accounts for a quarter of the group, and miscellaneous subtypes make up the remaining quarter. This preponderance of the passive-aggressive over the sociopathic is due partly to admission policies, which automatically excluded the more severe acting-out problems, and partly to our diagnostic inclinations. For example, we finally placed four patients in this category because a predominance of passive-aggressive behavioral patterns was obvious while the evidence for a suspected sexual perversion—homosexuality—was unclear. Four additional patients, who had mixtures of psychoneurotic symptoms and passive-aggressive patterns, were also put in this category.

Table 5. *Diagnosis of Personality Disorder by Subtype*

Personality Trait Disturbance	19
Passive-aggressive personality	
Sociopathic personality	9
Miscellaneous group	
Inadequate personality	3
Schizoid personality	2
Paranoid personality	1
Personality trait disturbance—other	2
Total	36

Personality Trait Disorder—Passive-Aggressive

In five patients out of the nineteen in this group the presence of a personality disorder on the initial interview was clear, but in only one was it possible to be confident about the specific subtype. This was a fourteen-year-old boy, with a passive-aggressive personality disorder, whose symptoms of persistent enuresis, asthma, thumb-sucking, and poor social life had begun in early childhood and persisted until the time of evaluation. The follow-up five years later confirmed the initial diagnostic impression. In three patients the difficulty was in differentiating a passive-aggressive subtype from a sociopathic, and in one a passive-aggressive subtype from schizophrenia, both of which problems have been illustrated in the previous chapter. Suffice it to say that time resolved all of these in favor of a passive-aggressive subtype.

In the remaining fourteen patients, for whom the diagnosis was in doubt on the initial interview, the difficulty, as already indicated, was in making a diagnosis of personality disorder in a clinical setting heavily colored by both psychoneurotic symptoms and conflict with a pathologic parent. These patients had no past history of psychoneurotic symptoms, but did have some rather mild manifestations of personality disorder: conduct disorder in school, dependency on the mother, obesity, enuresis, poor social adjustment, difficulties with self-assertion. Thus, present illnesses were strongly influenced by anxiety, depression, other psychoneurotic symptoms, and conflict with a pathologic parent. In addition, the present illness might contain some mild acting-out, difficulty in school, and psychophysiologic symptoms. A past history negative for psychoneurotic symptoms and positive for personality disorder manifestations combined with a present illness of intense psychoneurotic symptoms to indicate a diagnosis of a psychoneurosis or character neurosis. However, in all these cases the passage of time revealed the underlying personality disorder.

In retrospect, we feel that in some of these cases an alertness to the problem and greater persistence in eliciting the evidence for a personality disorder might have made an earlier diagnosis possible. In some, however, they would not have clarified the situation, and in a few, as we shall describe later, even five years later the diagnosis was still not clear. The practical usefulness of differentiating the psychoneurotic symptoms from an underlying personality disorder is indicated by the fact that in all probability the psychoneurotic symptoms or complaints would subside with or without treatment; treatment directed toward these symptoms, therefore, focuses the therapeutic effort on an aspect of the patient's problem that is going to disappear anyway, whereas without successful therapeutic intervention the underlying personality disorder will persist and cause future difficulty. (See Chapter 12.)

Sociopathic Personality

Two patients out of the nine in this group, presenting no diagnostic difficulty, had a consistent clinical picture in the present illness and in the past history of sociopathic personality; it was confirmed on follow-up five years later. The behavioral difficulties of these patients, beginning in early childhood, persisted in a consistent manner through adolescence to adulthood.

Another difficulty in four patients was to differentiate a sociopathic personality from a character neurosis. All had a past history of prominent psychoneurotic symptoms and mild manifestations of personality disorder which became intensified in the present illness. Since the manifestations of personality disorder had not reached the point of antisocial behavior, the diagnosis on the initial interview was difficult if not impossible to make. Nevertheless, in all four, subsequent events made the final diagnosis of sociopathic personality clear, suggesting that these patients may not have developed a sociopathic disorder till later in life. (See Chapter 7, pp. 71–72.)

A final difficulty in three patients was to differentiate this disorder from schizophrenia—in two because of multiple symptomatology and in one because of paranoid manifestations. Later developments confirmed a diagnosis of sociopathic personality, although in one, as shown in the second case example under Sociopath in Chapter 5, the paranoid elements raise the possibility that he is schizophrenic.

Thus we see three themes in the diagnosis of sociopathic personality. The first appears in those patients whose sociopathic behavior begins in early childhood and persists in a consistent manner through adolescence to adulthood, suggesting that their disorder is a continuous one. The second, in contrast, appears in those patients who may actually not develop their sociopathic disorder till later in life, perhaps during and after adolescence. In childhood they have prominent but mild psychoneurotic and personality disorder manifestations. In adolescence both of these intensify but there is still minimal evidence for a sociopathic disorder. As they grow to adulthood, however, the disorder takes a sociopathic direction. The last theme appears in those patients whose sociopathic disorder also begins early in life but contains schizophrenic elements which make it difficult to confirm the diagnosis until many, many years have passed.

These findings suggest that in many cases the disorder is impossible to diagnose at this time of life because the clinical picture is confused by either psychoneurotic coloring or schizophrenic elements and the sociopathic disorder has not fully asserted itself. However, cases in which sociopathic disorder appears in early childhood are easier to diagnose.

Inadequate Personality

In the three patients in this group the evidence on initial evaluation indicated a personality disorder, inadequate type, by reason of a history since childhood of unchanging dependency on the mother, unwillingness to grow up, and refusal to take responsibility. There was some doubt, however, due to the presence of mild acting-out. In all three the subsequent course confirmed the accuracy of the original diagnosis. The following case is a good example.

A fifteen-year-old girl, the fourth of four children, two of whom left school at an early age, had a long history of dependency on the mother, unwillingness to grow up, and refusal to do chores. In the year prior to admission, in the setting of attending an all-Negro school, she got into fights with her peers, was expelled, and was transferred to another school, which she refused to return to because she felt it was too strict. Past history revealed that the father left the mother when the patient was two, and from age three the patient continually talked about wanting a father and would go off with any man who smiled at her. At age twelve she would go into men's houses. On examination, she was unable to comprehend the abstractions, but her affect was normal and there was no thinking disorder. Our clinical impression varied from transient situational reaction to a personality disorder, either inadequate or sociopathic.

On follow-up at age twenty, it turned out that the patient had left school at fifteen and had about twenty jobs, resigning impulsively from one after another and drifting from job to job with long periods of remaining at home without work. She had a borderline IQ and expressed no future goals. She was obese, unkempt, and complained of constipation-diarrhea. She lived alone with her mother, on whom she remained excessively dependent, and was unwilling to assume any responsibility for herself. She dated but rarely, and entertained emotional fears about airplanes and tall buildings. She gave a history of one episode of hysterical blindness many years ago in school.

Follow-up five years later confirmed the diagnosis of inadequate personality through the persistence of the immaturity, unchanged dependence on the mother, obesity, poor work history, lack of involvement with men, and lack of future goals.

In retrospect, we feel that the presenting illness at age fifteen was but an interim episode in a progressive, uninterrupted history signalized by lack of personality development. Consequently, this dismal picture had been properly tagged on the initial interview. It is of interest that, as often happens with this type of patient, the childhood history is misleading in implying that no difficulty exists. For example, this patient as a child was obedient and compliant at home, did well in school, and was a teacher's pet. Not until later, when life required her to assume more responsibility, did her flagrant pathology become obvious.

Schizoid Personality

The two patients in this group, who showed the characteristic symptoms of a schizoid personality (see Chapter 5, pp. 53–55) that is, lifelong introversion, lack of assertiveness, social isolation, and tendencies toward autism—were both seen in treatment over a period of several years, one from age sixteen to twenty-one, the other from age seventeen to twenty-one. Neither developed schizophrenic symptomatology.

Residual Diagnostic Difficulties

Our journey now finished, the question arises, did we manage to circumvent the obstacles and reach the final destination in every instance? Did the passage of time resolve the diagnostic difficulties presented by every case? The diagnostic difficulties persisted in thirteen of the forty-one cases, or about one-third, because of the following factors: In eight, though we were confident of the diagnosis of a personality disorder, we continued to be unsure of the exact subtype because either the patients continued to show manifestations of more than one subtype, without clear evidence of which predominated (four cases), or they showed suggestive but inconclusive evidences that sexual perversion played a role in their personality disorder (four cases). In four the differential between a character neurosis and a personality disorder was not resolved by the passage of time, since the psychoneurotic symptoms did not abate and the manifestations of personality disorder did not become stronger. Therefore, five years later the psychoneurotic and personality disorder manifestations stood out equally and the diagnostic difficulties continued. In the last case, we had a reservation that the patient might eventually become schizophrenic. Thus, in only four, or 10 per cent of the cases, is there still significant diagnostic difficulty after five years.

Let us first consider the role of sexual perversion. In one case there was clear evidence from the present illness of a perversion (voyeurism) which persisted throughout the follow-up. In the other three cases we suspected either latent or unconscious homosexuality though the evidence was not sufficient to confirm this impression. In one case (Chapter 7, pp. 69–70) there was a history of homosexual play at age twelve and in both the present illness and the follow-up a lack of heterosexual interest or activity together with a great deal of denial of problems. A characteristic example of the role of unconscious homosexuality in a personality disorder is the following case.

The patient, a thirteen-year-old boy, gave a history since the age of nine of fainting spells occurring about once every three weeks for a year whenever he heard the word *blood* at school. This subsided from age ten until age twelve, when he refused to go to school because his peers teased him, tried to make him faint, and refused to play with him. However, at that time it was possible to persuade him to go back to school. At the time of admission he absolutely refused to consider attending school and had been truant for three months. An overindulgent mother had not started him in school until age seven because she liked to have him around the house. He had a passive, inadequate, distant father. Our initial impression was between a hysterical psychoneurosis and a personality disorder, passive-aggressive subtype.

On follow-up three years later, at age sixteen, the patient was picked up by the truant officer and brought to court for refusal to attend school. His anxiety had increased markedly, with restlessness, nail-biting, and nightmares of being stabbed in the back by an Oriental. He had become phobic, sleeping with his back against the wall with the doors locked, so that no one could sneak up and stab him, and closing the drapes when his mother was out of the house. He had also begun to act-out, stealing such things as records, soda, and candies, and he engaged in gang fights. Associated with this behavior were dreams and fears suggesting an underlying homosexual panic.

Under court duress at this time he started treatment with a male therapist. He participated well in the treatment, his fears diminished, and on second follow-up, at age nineteen, he gave a history of many brief jobs in the intervening years and had been working as a hospital orderly for four months. His symptomatology consisted of moderate anxiety, some hypochondriasis and still becoming dizzy, and occasionally fainting when blood was drawn. He had a possibly dependent relationship with a girl friend.

The diagnosis of a personality disorder appeared quite definite, with a thread of unconscious homosexuality running through the history. Starting with a passive, inadequate, distant father, who may himself have had unconscious homosexuality, and an overindulgent mother, the patient developed fainting spells at age nine, leading to refusal to go to school at age twelve to thirteen, perhaps to protect himself against homosexual impulses. As he became adolescent, he dreamed of being attacked by an Oriental and had fears of being stabbed in the back. Coincidentally he began to act-out aggressive impulses, also perhaps to defend himself against passive homosexuality. Identification with a male therapist enabled him to better control his homosexual impulses and perhaps to sublimate them into his occupation as a practical nurse. Further follow-up would be necessary to make the final diagnostic decision.

Let us turn now to the remaining difficulty of differentiating a character neurosis from a personality disorder, as shown by the example below.

The patient was a fifteen-year-old girl, referred by her pediatrician for obesity and conflict with her mother. The patient gave a history of anxiety and compulsive overeating when angry, with resultant obesity since the age of six, in a setting of marked conflict with her younger brother and with the mother, who nagged her about her eating habits. In recent years the patient had had other symptoms of anxiety, such as nail-biting, and nervousness and tension headaches. The mother reported that the patient had frequent colds and complained of fatigue. The patient had been unable to go to the public bathroom since she was a small child. Menarche occurred at age ten, without symptoms, and she had dated occasionally since that time. Schoolwork was average.

On examination, the patient was overweight, immature, anxious, and guarded; there were no other findings. The impression on the initial examination was either psychoneurosis with anxiety and obesity, or perhaps an underlying passive-dependent personality disorder.

When seen on follow-up at age twenty, the patient had been graduated from high school at seventeen, had gone to secretarial school for a year and night school to finish her stenography, but had lost interest and dropped out. She had been working as a secretary for several years and was recently promoted to supervisor of an office. Although she had lost 40 pounds, she was still 15 pounds overweight. She frequently began a new diet, only to give it up as soon as it became successful. She complained of occasional tension headaches and restlessness and was still in conflict with her mother, but tended to avoid her. She still reacted to the mother's nagging with rebellion, withdrawal, and overeating. She had been going with a boy whom she planned to marry, and she had an active social life and many outside interests.

On examination, she was anxious, moderately obese, guarded, and, according to her, without problems. The patient's clinical picture over the five years had altered in that its intensity was reduced, the conflict with the mother was handled by avoidance, she had lost some weight (though she was still overweight), and, while still anxious and restless, she functioned well at her place of employment and had a good social life. The final impression would be between character neurosis with anxiety and obesity, and a passive-dependent personality disorder. Some of the patient's difficulties may be masked by the fact that she is still living at home. Further follow-up would be necessary to clarify the diagnosis.

To summarize then: The diagnostic difficulties persisted, even after five years, because of several factors. First, though the personality disorder was definitely established, the passage of time did not clearly differentiate a subtype. Second, the role of unconscious homosexual factors in the personality disorder was not delineated. Third, the continuance of psychoneurotic manifestations at the same intensity as on the initial interview continued to confuse the diagnosis. On further reflection we can see that the residual diagnostic difficulty was most pressing only for the four patients whose clinical picture was a mixture of psychoneurosis and personality disorder. In the other nine, the diagnosis of personality disorder itself was certain, the doubt being only of the subtype.

CHAPTER 9

CHARACTER NEUROSIS

> Now when we had escaped the Rocks and dread
> Charybdis and Scylla, thereafter we soon came to the
> fair island of the god; where were the goodly kine,
> broad of brow, and the many brave flocks of Helios
> Hyperion.
>
> —Homer: *The Odyssey*,
> Book XII

JUST AS ULYSSES after passing Scylla and Charybdis, and Circe
came to the calm harbor of Trinacria, so we have negotiated the
rugged diagnostic journey of the personality disorders, to find that
the diagnostic dilemma in our last group contrasts with the dilemmas
of the other groups, as does a safe harbor with Scylla and Charybdis.
Since the patients in this final group showed neither the elements of
schizophrenia nor severe behavioral pathology, the grim, partially sub-
merged obstacles of diagnostic difficulty have been automatically
eliminated. A relatively safe harbor beckons: a psychoneurosis or a
character neurosis. In some (but far from all) respects, this safety is
an artifact, since we decided to forgo the differentiation between a
psychoneurosis and a character neurosis, feeling that it was still an
unsettled issue in psychiatry, that differentiation depended much
upon psychoanalytic data and insight and therefore was beyond the
scope of this study. Moreover, since the clinical pictures and outcome
for the patients now claiming our attention not only had much in
common but also differed significantly from those of patients with a
personality disorder or schizophrenia, we felt that they could readily
be studied as one separate group. The fact that we can eliminate
schizophrenia and personality disorder from consideration conveys a
wealth, not only of diagnostic meaning, but also of prognostic and
therapeutic optimism. We can automatically place these adolescents
in the diagnostic category whose outcome is universally the best of
the lot.

The clinical pictures of the patients with character neurosis had the
following features in common: a chief complaint of psychoneurotic
symptoms (anxiety, depression, phobias, and conversion symptoms);

an impairment of functioning limited to those areas affected by the psychoneurotic symptomatology; minimal evidence of developmental defects; much less intense dependency need, which appeared less frequently as a problem; minimal or absent behavioral pathology and school difficulties in the past; and little social difficulty. On examination, patients and parents showed much less denial and therefore for the most part were forthright and frank, and gave more reliable histories. Finally, later outcome was good. Three of the patients clearly had marked compulsive personality traits which, under the concepts of the American Psychiatric Association manual, would place them in the personality disorder category. We digressed from the APA practice because their clinical pictures had so little else in common with those in the personality disorder category. Similarly, in two other patients, it could be argued that their symptoms were conversion hysteria in the setting of a hysterical character neurosis.

To summarize then: We are clinically defining psychoneurosis or character neurosis as embracing those patients whose principal presenting problem was psychoneurotic symptoms uncomplicated by schizophrenia or personality disorder symptoms, who had neurotic traits in their character structure, and who had a relatively good outcome five years later.

The difference between the relative ease of diagnosis of this group and the dilemmas posed by the other is illustrated by the fact that we found no diagnostic difficulty on initial evaluation in seven of the eleven, or 63 per cent. The initial impression in each of the seven was confirmed on follow-up five years later. Three showed a clear clinical picture of a depression with marked compulsive personality traits, two showed evidence of conversion hysteria in hysterical character neuroses, one a mixed psychoneurosis with compulsive and hysterical features, and the seventh an anxiety neurosis. Further, of the four who did present a diagnostic problem, in one the differential diagnosis was between conversion hysteria and appendicitis, in another between conversion reaction and personality disorder, and in two between psychoneurosis and adjustment reaction of adolescence.

Cases Readily Diagnosed

We describe below two patients who presented no diagnostic difficulty initially and in whom the diagnosis was sustained throughout later developments. The first case illustrates a depression in a patient with marked compulsive personality traits.

A fourteen-year-old girl developed a depression a year and a half before admission, following the death of her father after a long illness. Three months prior to admission, she was rejected by a girl friend with whom she had formed a close relationship. Thereafter, she refused to go to school and threatened to commit suicide or to run away from home. When examined, she showed the classic features of a depression—early morning awakening, concentration difficulty, anorexia, easy fatigability. In addition, she was morose, hostile, resentful, and evasive, and she complained that her thinking and actions were definitely slowed. There was no affect or thinking disorder. She had a past history of being an excellent student, exceedingly conscientious about studying, but always had difficulty in making friends and participating in the usual social life of school. The mother reported that three years prior to admission the patient became moody and started to withdraw from the few friends she had, because of her humiliation when she failed to "make" a special class. The loss of the father, the classic symptoms of depression, and the compulsive personality characteristics clearly established the diagnosis of this patient.

Following the initial interview, the patient returned to school, and by age sixteen and a half her attendance had been perfect and she was number one in her class. Her menarche occurred shortly after the initial interview but was still irregular. She had mild tension headaches and occasional episodes of depression, insomnia, and nail-biting. She was popular, well liked, took things in her stride.

By the time she was nineteen, she had been graduated from high school with an "A" average, worked as a secretary during the summer, and started college in the fall but dropped out when she was overwhelmed by the amount of work. She again worked for six months as a secretary and then returned to college for another term, this time doing well.

At the time of the last interview, age nineteen, she was in her second semester of college with a less difficult schedule of courses. The patient complained of anxiety, palpitations, mild depression, and continued to be perfectionistic, meticulous, and obese. Life revolved around school, where she had to drive herself to study. She gave great attention to detail, was excessively neat, and berated herself if she did not meet her own high standards. She did homework every night and one day on the weekend. On dates every other week she engaged in necking and petting without intercourse. She had outside interests and activities and was ambivalent about her mother, sometimes feeling resentful.

The follow-up history confirmed the initial diagnosis of depression, from which the patient recovered rather readily. It also confirmed the presence of underlying compulsive personality traits with a characteristic history of mild depressive episodes, perfectionism, meticulousness, and attention to detail. Her compulsive need for superior performance, to do more than and better than her peers, resulted in her being overwhelmed by a college schedule which appeared insurmountable and doomed her to failure.

This clinical picture illustrated well the patients who had depression marked by compulsive personality traits, as well as one patient with a mixed psychoneurosis and the other with anxiety neurosis. The personality profile presented by these patients in adolescence is a classic one, seemingly little influenced—in form, at least—by adolescent turmoil, and it stays with them as they progress out of adolescence. This is a totally different story from the one we have been relating so far. The presenting clinical picture is definite and easily diagnosable; it does not vary much from that described in adults and does not change with the passage of time. Furthermore, these patients learn better to cope with the demands of growth into maturity and generally function better than patients in the other two groups.

The second case is one of a conversion reaction.

The patient was a fourteen-year-old girl, in the ninth grade, who three months prior to admission had a sudden attack of headache, weakness, and chills down the spine. She was sent home from school and soon developed numbness and shooting pains in the legs, for which she was hospitalized for one week. She had remained at home ever since (three months). As these symptoms abated, they were followed by dyspneic attacks and feelings of pressure in the chest and shoulders. At the time of the interview, the patient was bedridden and cared for by her mother. The past history was negative except for a history of anxiety and tension, school and social adjustment being good.

This patient gave a clear picture of acute conversion symptoms and there was no diagnostic difficulty. When seen on follow-up at age twenty-one, her symptoms were reported to have disappeared without treatment one year after the initial interview. During this year she had school instruction at home. She then returned to public school, was graduated from high school, and joined the Navy as a student nurse. She was recently discharged from the Navy, having been married for a year, and was now pregnant. She gave evidence of a complete recovery and denied any further difficulty.

Again we see a case with a typical picture of conversion hysteria which presented no diagnostic problem and had an uncomplicated resolution and an excellent outcome.

Cases Less Easily Diagnosed

We turn to the four cases where there was some diagnostic difficulty.

The first was that of a thirteen-year-old girl, who three months after the onset of her menarche developed continuous cramps and right lower quadrant pain. Medical evaluations were negative, as was the psychiatric evaluation, so that the diagnosis lay between appendicitis and conversion hysteria. Six months after the initial evaluation an appendectomy was performed. The patient has had no symptoms since, and when seen on final follow-up at the age of nineteen seemed to be making a good adjustment. Her initial complaint could have been the result of the appendicitis or it might have been a conversion reaction that preceded the appendicitis.

The next two patients were similar in that the differential problem was between an adjustment reaction of adolescence and a psychoneurosis. We present one case history.

A thirteen-year-old boy in the eighth grade was brought in by his mother with a report of homosexual play with a six-year-old male cousin and masturbating, both of which the patient denied. The mother was a controlling, domineering woman, separated from an alcoholic and irresponsible husband when the patient was seven. The patient was in marked conflict with three older siblings and resentful toward his mother for leaving his father and "causing him to get sick."

On examination, the patient was depressed and immature. He had some anxiety and tension, exhibited on testing as difficulty with abstractions. His school and social adjustment was good. The history disclosed no evidence of manifestations of personality disorder, so the impression was that of a psychoneurosis.

On second follow-up, when the patient was nineteen, it was found that he had left school at sixteen and had been working for two years as the manager of a shipping department. He was actively interested in music and was trying to organize a band. He showed mild compulsiveness about his band activities. He had been dating, with sexual intercourse, since age fifteen, had now been going steady for eight months and planned marriage. He was considerably more tolerant and understanding of his mother and reported no symptoms. The final diagnosis, though still somewhat tentative, was a psychoneurosis, with a reservation that he may at a later date show more difficulty.

We now describe the case which presented the most difficulty in this group, the differential problem being among a conversion reaction, epilepsy, and a personality disorder.

A sixteen-year-old boy, in the eleventh grade for the past six months, had been having (at a frequency of twice a month) convulsive-like seizures preceded by a gradual building up of irritation and characterized by uncontrollable movements of arms and legs, but without loss of consciousness or tonic or clonic spasms. After the first attack the patient grew increasingly anxious, restless, irritable, and depressed. "Everything disgusted me," he said. "I feel fed up." There was a history of fainting spells, some concentration difficulty, and a diminished quality of school performance.

On examination, he was depressed, with suicidal preoccupation, and he was troubled for fear his body form was not masculine enough. He reported that he slept with a knife under his pillow, played with the idea of suicide, and actually took a "large amount" of phenobarbital on one occasion. He was in marked conflict with his brother and his father, and when most irritated with them he would have a seizure-like attack. He once reported to his father an uncontrollable urge to beat up an old man. The electroencephalogram was class 4A with the typical spikes and waves consistent with epilepsy. The initial diagnostic impression was among a conversion reaction, epilepsy, and personality disorder. The seizures lacked the true epileptic criteria and seemed to be explained on a dynamic basis. However, the EEG indicated epilepsy. The patient's concern about his body's not being masculine enough and his expressed hostility to men suggested the possibility of unconscious homosexual factors.

On follow-up five years later, we found that within two years the seizures had stopped, and by age twenty-one, without medication, the patient had had no seizures for three years. He still had mild depression, which was less frequent and less intense, occasional tension headaches, and anxiety attacks (being mildly anxious in elevators and in crowds). He was a senior in college, planning to teach in high school after graduation, and had been going steady for two years with a girl with whom he was considering marriage. He had had sexual intercourse without difficulty. He was still preoccupied that his body structure might not be masculine enough and he wore a moustache. The father reported that he had stopped treatment twice because the doctor would not give him tests to rule out a pituitary tumor as causing feminization of his body.

There is no question that the possible unconscious homosexual and paranoid features in this patient's clinical picture may actually have constituted a personality disorder, but he was included in the category of psychoneurosis because of the prominence of his psychoneurotic symptoms, the minimal evidence of personality disorder, and the good outcome.

This group of psychoneuroses contrasts markedly with the other two categories in the almost complete freedom from schizophrenic elements or manifestations of personality disorder. The possibility that the diagnosis was based primarily on outcome is minimized because the clinical picture for the most part was that of a psychoneurotic syndrome which was readily diagnosed on the initial interview and did not show much variation with the passage of time. Again, where there is difficulty it is of an entirely different order from that found with schizophrenia and personality disorder.

Effect of Adolescent Turmoil

As we have noted before, the probable presence of adolescent turmoil in these patients does not complicate the clinical picture in such a way as to confuse the diagnosis. The patients in the category of psychoneurosis or character neurosis exhibit classic psychiatric syndromes which are consistent over time and are readily diagnosed when first seen. One might theorize that the effect of adolescent turmoil in these patients may be seen in their acute breakdown into psychoneurotic symptoms, such as conversion symptoms as well as anxiety and depression. But in all, as they grew older, with or without treatment, remissions were complete. Perhaps their personality structure is so rigidly organized that adolescent turmoil cannot produce the chaotic effect that it can in the loose, poorly organized personality structures of those with schizophrenia or personality disorder. It may cause an acute flare-up of psychoneurotic symptoms, which later subside as the patient, with age, gains better control of his adolescent turmoil.

At least in these cases, it would appear that where something is good it is all good. For example, the reports of the patients and parents are reliable, the clinical picture has a clear onset, its symptoms are very plain and well circumscribed, and there is a good later outcome. The indicated guideposts of our findings happily do lighten some of the clinician's burden, since he can approach these psychiatric illnesses in adolescence with a high degree of confidence that his diagnosis is accurate, his prognosis is reliable, and his patient *will* improve.

CHAPTER 10

EPILEPSY

I have had playmates, I have had companions,
In my days of childhood, in my joyful school-days.
All, all are gone, the old familiar faces.
—Charles Lamb: "Old Familiar
Faces"

T HIS CHAPTER WILL INCLUDE, in addition to the diagnostic difficulties and their resolution, the complete findings for the five patients with epilepsy. The diagnostic problems in these cases differed from those already described. First, there was less relevance to adolescence, since in three of the five cases both the behavior disorder and the epilepsy began in childhood; second, the history was adequate and the clinical picture clear; third, the source of most difficulty was in the decision as to the etiologic contribution to the clinical picture of each of the following: epilepsy, adolescent turmoil, conflict with a pathologic parent, a personality disorder, and physical defects such as mental deficiency.

Epilepsy and the concomitant reactions of the patient to his illness may have a profound influence on the development of a personality disorder, and contrariwise a personality disorder can intensify the symptoms of epilepsy. This is particularly well described by the following quotation from *Epilepsy and Convulsive Disorders in Children* by Edward M. Bridge [17]:

The child has been happy and in good health when suddenly a strange, terrifying feeling comes over him, the world goes black and he awakes to find himself in bed, the family excited and worried, a doctor beside him. Big words are spoken, medicine prescribed and he is made to stay in bed for the rest of the day with a dull headache and nothing to do. What happened, why all the excitement? He does not know, and something in the atmosphere gives him the feeling that he should not ask. The episode is never mentioned again, but for some reason he is now not allowed to eat meat, cabbage, peanuts or to play with the other boys. Every day he is asked how he feels, whether his bowels have moved, do his eyes trouble him? Perhaps he did have something bad, and everyone is wondering when it will come again.

It does come again with the same strange feeling. He tries to run to mother, tries to call for help, but the awful blackness is upon him. Again he wakes to family excitement, but this time the doctor is sewing up a cut on his forehead, or he finds his tongue very sore. How did he get these? When he fell in the faint. Too bad: He hopes that he will never get another one. But others follow, and he has them with increasing terror at the onset, and in between he is in more and more continual dread of them. Life becomes centered around these miserable spells, visits to doctors and hospitals, needles, medicines— everything that a boy wants to avoid. Furthermore, he is no longer allowed to go to school or to ride his bicycle. Why? A silly excuse for an answer. "All the other children do, why shouldn't I? She doesn't like me." The other children act strangely toward him now. One of them calls him "Fits" and the others laugh. "I'll beat him up for that."

Such situations tend to drive children into one of two general directions. The forceful robust child becomes the disagreeable domineering bully who covers up his dissatisfactions and insecurity by a hard crust. The less forceful, less vigorous child reacts with a sense of shame and disgrace, withdraws into his shell and leads a silent, solitary existence. He tries by overconscientious effort to create a favorable impression and a place for himself in the sun. Both types of child lack the insight and confidence necessary to reach a satisfactory balance. The attitudes of the family and physician add greatly to the potentialities of the situation.

Children frequently feel so much horror and dread at the approach of a seizure that a fear of dying comes over them. For years with each recurrent attack this expectation of dying may run through their minds. At the least suspicion of a warning aura they scream for help, run wildly to mother for protection, but sometimes realize that they fall down in the spell before help is available from anyone. They go into the seizure in a state of panic. The fact that recovery always occurs and usually without serious harm seems to make no impression until someone points it out to them. As time goes on the terror, inspired by warning sensations, develops on slighter and slighter provocation. Anticipation and dread become so intense that minor sensations from any part of the body may be interpreted as the dreaded aura. In circumstances sufficiently trying there is reason to believe that reactions of this kind may actually precipitate attacks. Certainly there can be no doubt from numerous observations made in the Epilepsy Clinic that seizures are more frequent and severe during periods when such emotional factors are known to be operating. Fear of death during the major seizures and continual dread of the next attack are very real difficulties in the minds of many children.

Reactions to the Handicaps

The child may also react with considerable violence to any restrictions placed upon him because of his illness and its treatment. He feels well between seizures and sees no reason for taking medicine, for maintaining a diet, or for limiting his play to games that would not cause injury if he should suddenly have an attack. He wants to be free, as others are, to enjoy himself and not to be a "sissy." The attitude is a natural and understandable one, and within limits is a commendable one. The difficulties arise most commonly in children who know nothing of what goes on during a seizure, of the possible outcome of the disease, or of the reasons for the various recommendations and restrictions that have been placed on them. Too often the situation is handled entirely between doctor and family, the child being simply a pawn, expected to do as he is told.

There is also wide variation in the degree and intensity of personality disorders in children with epilepsy. Bridge (p. 162) reports in a study of 742 children with epilepsy that 54 per cent had no personality disorder, 37 per cent had a mild or moderate personality disorder, and 9 per cent had a severe personality disorder. All our patients had personality disorders, four of them severe. On initial evaluation it was impossible to make more than an educated guess as to the relative influence of each of the etiologic factors, since the clinical picture was a combination of them all. However, in a few, as time passed, behavior improved and some of the etiologic factors ameliorated, and it became clearer in retrospect which had played the predominant role —for example, such changes as control of convulsions, decrease in conflict with parent, getting older and therefore perhaps getting better control of adolescent turmoil.

There were two clinical types of these five patients. (1) Three patients had a past history from childhood of epilepsy, conflict with parent, and a personality disorder, and all of their symptoms became aggravated in adolescence. (2) Two patients had a history from childhood of a personality disorder, but their epilepsy began in early adolescence. Let us emphasize several additional points, which will be brought out in the cases described below. The adolescent growth process seemed to intensify a condition which had existed from early childhood. For example, contrary to the finding for personality disorder, all of the patients when first seen were between thirteen and fourteen years old. A long history of severe difficulty, together with a presenting clinical picture that was also dramatically severe, did not necessarily predict a poor outcome. The problems in family relationships were essentially the same as those described in Chapter 4. Likewise, as described in Chapter 11, these patients did not grow out of their difficulties, though one improved remarkably. Finally, symptom variations were somewhat different from those described in Chapter 11: In three cases, both acting-out and depression decreased with the passage of time, while in a fourth acting-out persisted and in a fifth depression came to the fore.

Epilepsy Beginning in Childhood

The first case illustrates the etiologic mixture of three factors: epilepsy, personality disorder, and conflict with the parent. The latter element could not be clarified until later, when it was obvious that as the parents had lifted their restrictions, not only had their conflict with the patient subsided, but the patient's acting out had ceased and his depression had abated; however, his hostility was then channeled into intense phobic symptomatology which previously had been mild.

A thirteen-and-a-half-year-old boy gave a history of nervousness, anxiety, stuttering, and poor social life since childhood. Five years prior to admission, at the age of nine, following the birth of his sister, he had the onset of grand mal epilepsy. At this time all of his symptoms worsened, and he developed increasingly uncontrollable hostility to a domineering and pathologic mother, as well as toward his teachers. His behavior was marked by impulsiveness and dramatic suicidal threats during arguments. He would eat voraciously, especially when disciplinary measures were enforced, and consequently he was obese. He bit his nails and complained of constant fatigue, and his teachers reported decreased school performance with difficulty in comprehension. The mother, on the one hand, was overindulgent to the point of making a baby of her son, and she was fearful that his epilepsy severely damaged his chances in life. On the other hand, she was critical, nagging, demanding, and restrictive. Both parents, however, denied that they or the patient had any emotional problems.

This patient presented a minimum of diagnostic difficulty, since he clearly had a personality disorder with epilepsy. The principal question was an etiologic one—the relative contribution to his present illness of epilepsy, the personality disorder, conflict with the patho-logic mother, or adolescent turmoil. Since this condition became worse after the onset of the epilepsy at age nine, it would seem that adolescent turmoil had an exacerbating influence, such as increasing the strength of the instinctual forces with which the patient had to cope. These forces were further intensified by the conflict with the mother at the same time that his capacity to handle his problems was being weakened by both the epilepsy and the beginning of adolescence. Small wonder that his condition became worse.

When seen on follow-up, the patient, then age eighteen, presented essentially the same clinical picture. His parents had refused his request to go to the clinic for treatment, and he had left school. He was anxious and depressed, had great trouble controlling his hostility, and had made several suicidal attempts which seemed to be more gesture than genuine. He had had no grand mal seizures in three years, possibly in four, but was having petit mal seizures about five times a month. Despite these symptoms he was able to hold a job as a stock clerk.

When he was seen on second follow-up, at the age of nineteen, his parents, feeling less burdened by their responsibility, had lifted their restrictions and the patient's depression and hostility had decreased markedly. He had, however, become intensely phobic, with nail-biting and sleep difficulty. His stuttering and obesity had remained. Although he took his medicine, he had had two convulsions in the last year. His life was extremely restricted by his phobias and his epilepsy. He took an early subway train in the morning to avoid crowds and, to avoid walking on the sidewalk at night, did not go out socially. Though he was doing well at work, where he had received several raises, he had few interests or outside activities. He remained dependent on his mother and had no dates with girls.

The five-year picture clarified the initial clinical impression, in that the acting-out in retrospect seemed to be related to all the etiologic factors—adolescent turmoil, pathologic parent, epilepsy, and personality disorder. The acting-out diminished markedly as he got older and as the parents became less restrictive. Although able to work, and not suffering so much from depression, he was nevertheless not handling his hostility successfully through his various phobias, which in themselves produced moderate impairment. Clearly this patient did not grow out of his difficulties.

The next patient, with a similar history of epilepsy and the symptomatology of a personality disorder from early childhood, illustrates an unchanging, consistent clinical picture right through from age three to age nineteen.

This fourteen-year-old girl, in the eighth grade, was having grand mal convulsions pre- and postmenstrually, about once or twice a month, although being treated with Dilantin and phenobarbital. She was anxious and hypochondriacal and had a poor social life and so much difficulty in school that she had to repeat the fifth grade. The patient had recently become preoccupied with boys and their sexual curiosity.

The mother denied the presence of any problems except epilepsy and appeared to be subtly rejecting, frequently showing irritation at the patient's preoccupation with her health and her affectionate outbursts. She hinted that she felt the patient was always complaining about herself and she nagged the patient about her slowness and her lack of conformity. As a reaction-formation, the mother reminded herself to give the patient affection and said many things she did not feel in an effort to be encouraging. The father, on the other hand, favored the patient, "adored her," and when drunk would not be verbally abusive to her as he was to the mother and sister. The patient took care of him, made him special coffee, and felt more at ease with him than with her mother.

On examination, she was extremely tense, anxious, restless, and depressed. She showed poor concentration, marked comprehension difficulty, but no affect or thinking disorder. She reported recurrent stomach pains since the age of seven. In addition, she was apathetic, with slurred speech, and in early adolescence expressed her rebellion against her mother by not taking medicine. The diagnostic impression on the initial interview was a personality disorder, inadequate type, with low IQ, epilepsy, anxiety, and depression. Except for her concern about boys and their sexual curiosity and increased conflict with her father, there was little evidence that adolescent turmoil was playing a role in this case.

The initial diagnostic impression was confirmed by the follow-up. When seen at the age of nineteen, the patient was in essentially the same condition. She had been graduated from high school four months before the interview, barely passing the general course. She was then attending a business school, having previously left another because of disagreements with one of the teachers. She was taking Dilantin and phenobarbital, as well as two other medicines, and had had no grand mal seizures for two and a half years, but she had petit mal six or seven times a day. She got very depressed when the attacks occurred frequently and, overcome by her feelings of futility, cried. She was still anxious, still restless on going to bed; she had difficulty in learning and during the day "felt groggy prior to medication." She had attacks of palpitation and dizziness. Her relationship with her father continued to deteriorate and her conflict with him remained. Social life was practically nil. Although she dated rarely, for one year at age sixteen she had gone steady with a boy, petting but having no other sexual experience. On examination, she was apathetic, her thinking was slowed, she appeared groggy, and the affect was blunted. There was poor comprehension, concentration difficulty, but no affect or thinking disorder. Her impairment of functioning was considered moderate.

As this patient got older, the chief change was the addition of greater anxiety, and depression with feelings of futility. Clearly, she seemed to be suffering equally from the effects of the conflict with her mother and the impairment of her functioning due to the petit mal seizures, and perhaps to a less extent from adolescent turmoil. In addition, the low IQ further burdened her efforts to struggle with these manifold problems.

The next case illustrates how a history since early childhood of manifestations of personality disorder along with epilepsy, together with a flagrant presenting clinical picture, does not necessarily indicate a poor outcome.

A thirteen-and-a-half-year-old girl had had petit mal epilepsy, rebelliousness, and severe conflict with her mother since age five, forgetting to take her medicine and in the last two months running away from home. Both her performance in school and her social life were poor. She had been placed in a foster home at age two and a half by her mother, whom the foster home mother described as "unfit." The patient had poor understanding and comprehension and had had recurrent failures in school, without, however, having had to repeat a grade. She had one sister who was mentally retarded.

On examination, she was apathetic, evasive, vague, and immature. She had four petit mal attacks during the interview. Her affect was blunted, she had concentration difficulty, and her comprehension of abstractions was poor. Her IQ was 85, and the EEG tracings were consistent with a convulsive disorder. Again the elements of the clinical picture are clearly those of personality disorder, epilepsy, mental deficiency, and conflict with a pathologic mother. The problem is to evaluate the relative or combined influences of each of these factors. The long history of severe difficulty prior to adolescence suggests that adolescent turmoil exerted at most an exacerbating influence. This patient's later course, described below—and better than anticipated— tends to clarify the relative contribution of each of the diagnostic factors to her clinical picture.

For six months, at age fourteen and again at age fifteen, the patient was hospitalized for unmanageable behavior. However, when seen on second follow-up, the patient, who was then nineteen, had married a Spanish man at the age of sixteen and her disturbance of conduct had disappeared. She had a four-month-old son, whom she cared for, a good relationship with her husband, and only occasional epileptic seizures since the birth of her child, although she had stopped taking her medicine. Most of the acting-out which had been in existence before marriage had disappeared. Her main symptomatology consisted of headaches, anxiety, nightmares, mild phobias, and menstrual cramps. Although still immature and dependent on her husband, she managed well. Her resentment toward her mother and the difficulties with her siblings had also subsided. On examination, though her affect was blunted, she was spontaneous and not suspicious or guarded. She was also obese and fearful of cemeteries and airplanes. Both the acting-out and the depression were absent.

The five-year history suggests that on the initial evaluation the most important factors in the patient's behavior were in all probability the low IQ, epilepsy, the conflict with the pathologic mother, and finally the increase in the instinctual forces with adolescence. Her low IQ and her epilepsy made functioning in school difficult. Her poor emotional control led to impulsive acting-out and severe conflict with her mother. As the patient grew older and as she formed a satisfactory though dependent relationship with a man, her acting-out subsided, but she developed anxiety, phobias, and psychophysiologic symptoms. However, she lives in a restricted environment with little social life and few other demands, and although she has epileptic seizures she is not on any medication. Though she is functioning quite adequately now, the feeling persists that she would not respond too well to stress, particularly if it involved conflict with her husband. A final diagnosis would be a personality disorder, passive-dependent type, with epilepsy and dull-normal IQ.

Epilepsy Beginning in Adolescence

We turn now to the second clinical type, personality disorder, with symptoms from early childhood and the onset of epilepsy in early adolescence. One patient, as the history might suggest, had a very poor outcome, while the other did well. The first patient had a long history of sociopathic-like behavior from early childhood, with convulsions beginning in early adolescence. The later course suggests that the epilepsy was a minimal influence in the sociopathic personality disorder, and it was the latter which was primarily responsible for his clinical picture.

A thirteen-and-a-half-year-old boy gave a history since age seven of stealing, lying, temper tantrums, immaturity, and enuresis. He had had poliomyelitis at age five, with some residual impairment in his left arm, and an operation for inguinal hernia at age seven. He was a food faddist and would not eat anything colored red. His school performance was adequate, but it was difficult for him to be friendly with his peers, so he played with younger friends. The father was overseas when the patient was born, returned home when he was five, divorced the mother when he was six, remarried, and rarely saw the patient. He was described as quiet, withdrawn, selfish, and irresponsible. The mother, trying to be both mother and father to the patient, tended to nag about his hours of returning home and where he had been. He would resent her nagging and not tell her where he was going, and as he grew older she gradually became quite disinterested.

On examination, the patient denied having any problems, and there was no affect or thinking disorder. Most of the history had to be obtained from the mother. In the last six months, since the beginning of the epilepsy, the patient had been picked up by the police twice for attempting to molest a younger girl. The influence of adolescent turmoil seemed to be to add to the difficulty in controlling aggressive and sexual impulses. The diagnostic impression at that time was a developing sociopathic personality.

In the next two years the patient's condition seemed to be veering away from a sociopathic direction. When seen at age sixteen, he was in the tenth grade. On examination, he again showed marked denial of any problems and some evidence of perfectionism. There had been no recurrence of convulsions, enuresis had disappeared, and the sexual acts had not been repeated. He stole occasionally from his mother, lied at times, and often purposefully behaved so as to provoke his mother, with whom he was in perpetual conflict. His school record, however, was excellent. The patient wanted to attend Harvard University and was much interested in the several clubs he belonged to at school. His arm was in a cast following a recent operation to relieve limitation of its motion.

On second follow-up the patient was eighteen, but we could see his mother only. She reported that in the second term of his senior year his behavior began to get worse. There were increased incidents of lying and temper outbursts, truancy, withdrawal, and moodiness. He became careless in personal hygiene, where before he had been meticulous, neat, and tidy. He gambled, ran up debts, received a suspended sentence for forging a check, and was indicted for breaking and entering a house and sent to a penitentiary. His mother did not visit him in prison, did not remember the term of his sentence, did not see him before he left, nor did this relationship change over the years, except that as the patient acted-out more he became more friendly with his father. There was also the possibility that he had been taking narcotics.

A salient feature of this story is the remarkable improvement between age thirteen and age fifteen, which, however, must remain suspect in view of the patient's extensive denial of having problems. In contrast to the other cases, as he got older and theoretically gained better control of his adolescent turmoil and as his convulsions disappeared, his acting-out did not lessen but actually flagrantly worsened and clinched the final diagnosis: sociopath.

The fifth and last case illustrates a patient with manifestations of personality disorder from early childhood of severe difficulty in controlling aggressive impulses, who in early adolescence came into severe conflict with his twin sister (he was physically underdeveloped and his sister was a few inches taller than he) and developed epilepsy. However, on follow-up, with control of his epilepsy and good physical development, he showed a remarkably good outcome.

A thirteen-year-old boy had a lifelong history of restlessness, of temper tantrums, and of hitting his mother when angry since age six. In spite of recurrent depressions and unruly conduct in school, he managed to do passing work. Belligerent with his peers, he had few friends. The father, more pathologic than the mother, was described as tense, nervous, irritable, possibly paranoid. All these difficulties were projected upon his wife, and he was in equally severe conflict with his workers as well, all of which he denied. He "hollered" at the children and was domineering and opinionated and occasionally impulsive. It was further stated that he "never understands anything, never believes people, has no sympathy" and worked all the time. He had no time for the patient. He socialized by himself and encouraged the mother to go out on her own. The mother, however, was compulsive, neat, meticulous, and overindulgent of her son. A year prior to admission, the patient's symptoms worsened in the setting of bitter rivalry with his twin sister, who had grown much taller than he. In one fit of anger he threatened to stick a knife into her. Several months before examination, the onset of grand mal seizures occurred. There was also a past history of head injury at the age of five.

On examination, he was immature, physically undeveloped, evasive, and guarded, but his affect was normal. There was no thinking disorder but he had a concentration difficulty. He was preoccupied with his trouble in controlling his temper. The differential diagnosis was between an organic behavior disorder, perhaps due to cerebral injury and epilepsy, and a personality disorder. The adolescent growth process seemed to play a role in that, at age thirteen in rivalry with his sister, the patient's symptoms were aggravated, with increasing difficulty in controlling aggressive impulses.

This patient's follow-up course was in marked contrast to that of the previous four. When seen at age fifteen, he had grown 5 inches in the two-year period, had become taller than his sister, and had had no seizures, these having been almost immediately controlled with Dilantin. All of his dramatic outbursts of anger had disappeared. He was able to control his temper better, he performed better and behaved acceptably in school, and his social life was now more interesting. He was less hostile toward his sister. The only persistent symptomatology consisted of anxiety, mild fears and some nightmares, and some depression occasioned by his preoccupation with the recurrent fights between his mother and father. On examination, his affect was normal and he had no thinking disorder.

When seen on second follow-up at age eighteen, he had continued to improve. He was attending college part time and working part time, and doing well in both activities. He had an active social life, many interests in outdoor activities—swimming, boating, diving, bowling, baseball—and he was dating, with little sexual activity other than kissing. He had attempted to go steady twice without success. He felt close to his mother, but distant and angry with his domineering, rejecting father. Moderate levels of anxiety persisted, but he no longer suffered from phobias. He had occasional mild depression when his parents fought. Psychiatric examination was normal. In the interim period he had handled well the death of his maternal grandmother, for whom he had a warm affection. There remained some hints of dependency on his mother and vagueness about future goals.

The original intense belligerence of the acting-out and its long history, together with the residual immaturities at age eighteen, suggest a personality disorder as the most likely diagnosis. On the other hand, the dramatic improvement following control of the epilepsy and his growing taller as he grew older argues strongly that both the epilepsy and adolescent turmoil were also powerful factors in the presenting illness. A few more years' follow-up would help to clinch the diagnosis and allow us to say with more conviction that this exceptional patient had grown out of his difficulties.

The course of this case, as of the first and third cases under Epilepsy Beginning in Childhood, suggests the presence of a somewhat reliable prognostic factor in the presenting clinical picture: an environmental precipitating stress which increased the patient's hostility. For example, in this last case the lack of physical development and the rivalry with the taller sister represented an unbearable threat to an adolescent boy. In the previous case the conflict with the mother and in the first case the birth of a sister and the conflict with the mother, who was fearful and restrictive, were sources of serious stress. These environmental precipitating factors, then, add almost an overload of hostility, which occasions so flagrant a clinical picture of depression and acting-out that a poor prognosis may well be suggested. However, with control of the epilepsy and elimination of the environmental precipitating factors—such as the growing taller of this last patient, escaping from the mother by leaving home and marriage for patient three, the lifting of parental restrictions for patient one—came dramatic improvement. Depression and acting-out subsided, and the patients managed to function better, though still somewhat impaired by anxiety and phobic symptoms.

In addition, it would appear that focus on their histories would immediately lead to a poor prognosis, since in all five of these patients with epilepsy the history was poor. Yet closer study of the last two cases reveals a significant prognostic difference. The patient whose acting-out behavior was antisocial showed much denial, while the other patient, though having great difficulty in controlling his hostility, exhibited no antisocial behavior and, far from denying his problems, was actually quite concerned about gaining control.

To summarize: Adolescent turmoil does not seem to contribute anything unique to the problems involved in the diagnosis of epilepsy except as it intensifies or aggravates a preexistent condition. The diagnostic problem in adolescence is essentially the same as in childhood, i.e., to evaluate the influence of epilepsy on the personality disorder or, conversely, the influence of personality disorder on the epilepsy. There is the additional factor of precipitating environmental stress. We found that the initial clinical pictures were a mixture of these reciprocal forces, which were impossible to separate at the time. However, follow-up did make it possible to separate one or more as the predominant force in the presenting clinical picture. One patient improved so markedly in his behavior as to permit at least a tentative claim that he had grown out of his difficulties. On the other hand, for another patient, in the penitentiary at second follow-up, the outlook for his ever coping with his problems was grim indeed. Whereas the other three clearly did not grow out of their difficulties, they did, as is described in Chapter 12, manage to make some fairly acceptable adjustment to them.

SECTION IV
CLINICAL OUTCOME

CHAPTER 11

SYMPTOM PATTERN FLUCTUATIONS

> Tension and release followed one another deter-
> mined by manifold influences, forever assuming new
> forms, but remaining without a pivot and without
> cumulative substance.
> —Martin Buber: *Mein Weg zum
> Chassidismus* (*Memoirs of My
> People*)

IT HAS BEEN SUGGESTED (see Chapter 1, particularly the comments of Eissler [21] and Josselyn [39]) that adolescent turmoil causes a patient's clinical picture not only to shift from one diagnostic category to another but also to show a great deal of change and flux in symptom patterns within a diagnostic category. In Chapters 5 through 10, it was demonstrated that some patients, rather than shifting from one diagnostic category to another, tended over the course of time to differentiate more clearly into the clinical pictures usually associated with each diagnostic category. This chapter, dealing with the second part of the theory, symptom pattern changes within a diagnostic category, asks: How do symptom patterns fluctuate as these patients pass through adolescence? The answer to this question was most significant for the symptom patterns of depression and act-ing-out, which therefore form a second principal theme.

Since symptomatology can theoretically shift within an hour or a day as well as over longer periods, the best evidence for variation in symptom pattern would be that derived from patients seen frequently in treatment over long periods of time, permitting observation of sud-den transient shifts in symptomatology which might be missed by in-terviews spaced at greater intervals. The complexity of the problem is indicated by the fact that even under these circumstances it is necessary to account for the effect of treatment on the observed shift in symptom patterns. All the patients were interviewed at three points in time: initially at the age of sixteen, two and a half years later at age eighteen and a half, and five years later at age twenty-one—the chron-ological end of adolescence. Therefore, our findings can be viewed as three cross sections rather than as an ongoing record derived from a treatment setting. However, thirty of the forty-two patients treated were seen at the Payne Whitney Clinic (from periods ranging from a few months to, in some cases, several years), and retrospective analysis of the records of these thirty led to the same conclusions as were found on the cross-sectional evaluation of the seventy-two patients. This material was not included here as it was not part of the methodology.

When we looked for the persistence of symptom patterns (see Chapter 2) from one interview to the next, we found that some disappeared, more persisted at both subclinical and clinical levels of intensity, and one, depression, not only persisted but actually appeared in an increasing number of patients with the passage of time. The findings for the symptom patterns of depression and acting-out are presented in tables with illustrative case examples. The findings for the other symptom patterns—anxiety, conversion, phobic, obsessive-compulsive, hypochondriacal, and psychophysiologic (migraine and asthma)—are presented descriptively. Also included are several findings on examination such as concentration difficulty, blunted affect, and obesity, and a behavioral manifestation of psychopathology—poor socialization.

Depression

Table 6 presents the distribution of the symptom pattern of depression in percentage of patients in each diagnostic category on each interview.

Observing first the total percentage of patients with the symptom pattern of depression, we note that this figure remains about the same from initial interview to first follow-up (34.7 per cent to 32.3 per cent) but shows a dramatic increase from first follow-up to second follow-up (32.3 per cent to 51.4 per cent). When we turn next to the diagnostic categories, we note that most of this increase is due to patients with personality disorder, from 38.4 per cent on first follow-up to 55.8 per cent on second follow-up, since there is little change in those with schizophrenia over the three interviews, and those with psychoneurosis show a marked drop on first follow-up which is later restored by second follow-up. This increase, which occurred almost exclusively in those with sociopathic and passive-aggressive disorders, was further demonstrated by the fact that ten of the twelve patients depressed on initial interview remained depressed on second follow-up, and fourteen additional patients not depressed on initial interview were depressed on second follow-up. There were also more on follow-up with the symptom of suicidal preoccupation (three on initial, five on follow-up). Thus depression strikingly increased as these patients grew out of adolescence.

Table 6.   Symptom Pattern by Diagnosis:
Depression Symptom Pattern

Diagnosis	Initial		First Follow-up		Second Follow-up	
	Total No. of Pts.	Sx.P.* (%)	Total No. of Pts.	Sx.P.* (%)	Total No. of Pts.	Sx.P.* (%)
Personality disorder	43	27.9	39	38.4	43	55.8
Schizophrenia	18	44.0	16	38.0	18	50.0
Psychoneurosis	11	45.5	10	0	11	36.4
Total	72	(34.7)	65†	(32.3)	72	(51.4)

* Sx.P. = symptom pattern
† Sixty-five patients were seen on both initial and first follow-up, whereas seventy-two were seen on initial and second follow-up.

Why do patients with a personality disorder show such a rise in depression between ages eighteen and twenty-one, when, theoretically, their adolescent turmoil should be subsiding? To investigate this question, we clinically reviewed all the material on twenty-four patients found to be depressed on second follow-up. It was our impression that the factor that seemed to exert the most formative influence on the course and development of their psychiatric illness, as they progressed through and emerged from their adolescent years, was not in the subsidence of adolescent turmoil but in an increasing frustration arising from inability to cope with the demands of adult life adjustment. As adult life placed greater strain on their meager adaptive capacities, they were less able to cope with their environment, their dependent needs became more frustrated, and either a previously existent depression came to the fore or they developed a depression for the first time.

The case history in Chapter 7, pages 73–74, is a good example. This patient's fights with her husband, dating from the beginning of the marriage, had worsened to the point of physical combat, and the patient had become markedly depressed with feelings of futility and hopelessness. She had made one suicidal attempt, and had tried self-mutilation by pushing her hand through a window.

This brief case illustrates well the theme of the development of depression in personality disorder. On initial evaluation it either played a minor role in the clinical picture or actually remained in the wings, but by the time of the follow-up interview, with ever increasing difficulties in coping with the environment, it came to have a major role or even took over the center stage.

Acting-Out

Table 7 presents the percentage of patients with the symptom pattern of acting-out in each diagnostic category at each interview.

Table 7. Symptom Pattern by Diagnosis: Acting-Out Symptom Pattern

Diagnosis	Initial		First Follow-up		Second Follow-up	
	Total No. of Pts.	Sx.P. (%)	Total No. of Pts.	Sx.P. (%)	Total No. of Pts.	Sx.P. (%)
Personality disorder	43	55.8	39	69.2	43	48.8
Schizophrenia	18	50.0	16	31.2	18	31.2
Psychoneurosis	11	9.1	10	0	11	0
Total	72	(47.2)	65*	(33.8)	72	(36.1)

* Sixty-five patients were seen on both initial and first follow-up, whereas seventy-two were seen on initial and second follow-up.

First we note that about one-half of the patients have this symptom pattern and that it decreases by about one-third by first follow-up and stays at that level to second follow-up. So acting-out becomes somewhat less common from sixteen to eighteen, then persists at that level from eighteen to twenty-one. Examination of the diagnostic categories reveals little acting-out in those with psychoneurosis, and in those with schizophrenia there is the same trend as in the total group, i.e., a decrease of one-third by first follow-up, unchanged through second follow-up. Those in the personality disorder category show approximately the same level throughout the three interviews, one-half of the patients displaying acting-out as a symptom pattern. The persistence of this symptom pattern in patients with personality disorder is indicated by the fact that two-thirds of those with acting-out on initial interview still have it on second follow-up. To further illuminate the symptom pattern of acting-out in these patients we studied the component symptoms (see Chapter 2) and found that stealing remained about the same (seven on initial interview, five on follow-up), as did temper outbursts (twelve on initial interview and fifteen on follow-up). A few had the symptoms of general negativism or physical attacks on parents or siblings on initial interview, and these disappeared on second follow-up. There was an increase in antisocial behavior (three initially to seven at second follow-up) and in sexual acting-out (five initially to nine at follow-up). The sociopathic subcategory had more with antisocial behavior: four with histories of arrests, two with alcoholism, three with drug addiction, and one with a history of rape.

These findings indicate that in the personality disorders, though the incidence of acting-out does not increase, it is still just as persistent a symptom pattern as depression over the course of time; and that in sociopaths, as the patient gets older, the acting-out takes a more antisocial direction.

The question that arises here is not why the acting-out persists, since we would expect it to do so in patients with a personality disorder, but how the form of the acting-out varies over time. Does it appear in the same way after adolescence as during adolescence? To answer this question, we clinically reviewed the twenty-one patients with acting-out on second follow-up. The first theme—that of progressively more antisocial acting-out—has already been indicated and will not be elaborated on since it is commonly seen by most clinicians. The theme of directly translating the conflict with and acting-out against the parent to conflict with acting-out against the environment was illustrated in the first case history in Chapter 7. We will finally demonstrate here a last theme, that when the patient's acting-out symptom pattern persists, he is able to adjust with little symptomatology since his environment is conducive to the acting-out.

The patient was a seventeen-year-old high school senior, referred to our clinic because of his failures in school. Since age eleven, when the parents were mistakenly informed that the patient had an IQ of 140 and placed great pressure on him to achieve in school, he had underachieved and failed a subject on each report card. He had continued to fail a subject every year since entering high school. He resented the parental pressure and expressed his feelings by not applying himself to his studies. The parents reported a past history of restlessness and attention-getting behavior in school. In addition, the last few years the patient's father had been ill with diabetes and shown less interest in his son. Despite his difficulties, the patient was active in extracurricular activities, such as the YMCA, clubs, and the student organization. He was manager of the football team.

On examination, the patient was tall, looked older than his age, had great verbal facility, spoke quite easily, and, though restless, related well to the examiner. There was some anxiety, evasiveness, and concentration difficulty, but no thinking disorder.

At age twenty, the patient presented essentially the same picture. He managed to graduate from high school by taking extra courses. He attended college and then flunked out, still rebelling against his parents' pressure. After dropping out of college he served six months in the Coast Guard, whereupon he resumed college and again flunked out. At this point he reported that the parents' pressure was still present, but he denied feeling rebellious, wanted to learn but was not interested in working, and wanted to leave home as soon as possible. He was going steady with a girl, with whom he was in great conflict because she was not responsive to his inordinate sexual demands. He reported being under constant pressure for sexual release, for which he resorted to frequent masturbation. He felt that his mother, who stopped her education after high school, always wanted him to go to college to fulfill her own frustrated desires.

When seen on final follow-up, at the age of twenty-two, the patient was 6 feet 1 inch tall, weighed 210 pounds, and was well dressed, cooperative, friendly, glib, and loquacious. He had worked his way up in the television industry from clerical worker to an assistant television producer. He spoke of his ambition and of his sexual prowess as evidenced by many girl friends and frequent sexual experiences. He seemed to emphasize and boast of his masculinity as if to compensate for his feelings of inadequacy. He gave an impression of glibness, superficiality, and manipulativeness. His symptomatology consisted of obesity and occasional smoking of marajuana. Despite this report of successful adjustment, some doubt remains as to its completeness and stability. The patient loves his work and is evidently quite successful at it; at the same time, however, he is in the Coast Guard Reserve and must attend meetings once a week. Here he has come into great conflict with his superior officer, and this he acts-out to such an extent that he is in danger of losing his job by being redrafted into the Coast Guard as a punitive measure for his insubordination. The final impression is that he has a sociopathic personality and is narcissistic and manipulative with a shallow affect and much denial of underlying problems. This suggests that should he be required to function in an environment other than his present optimal one he would surely seem to be headed toward a great deal more difficulty.

Anxiety, Conversion, Phobic, Obsessive-Compulsive, Hypochondriacal, and Psychophysiologic Symptom Patterns

The findings for these symptom patterns are presented descriptively rather than in tabular form.

The anxiety symptom pattern was, as might be expected, common on initial interview and both follow-ups (initial interview, 73.6 per cent; first follow-up, 67 per cent; and second follow-up, 76.4 per cent). Eighty per cent of the patients with anxiety on initial interview were found to have this symptom pattern on second follow-up.

Conversion symptom patterns were few in number (six) and of great clinical intensity and disappeared in all but one patient within a year.

There were six patients with phobic symptom patterns on initial evaluation, four at a clinical level of intensity and two subclinical. In two of the former it persisted at a clinical level of intensity, while in the other four it remained, but at a subclinical level. Ten additional patients, not found to have a phobic symptom pattern initially, did have it on second follow-up—in nine to a subclinical degree and in one to a clinical degree. The phobic pattern, like the conversion pattern, was not frequent and when present was clinically intense, improved with time, but then persisted at a subclinical level.

Obsessive-compulsive symptoms* and compulsive character traits† were analyzed together. Five patients with obsessive-compulsive symptoms initially continued to show them at a reduced level of intensity on follow-up. Three patients initially were found to have compulsive

---

* Obsessive thoughts, usually of a sexual or aggressive nature, or compulsive behavior, such as compulsive rituals or compulsive eating.

† Obsessive ruminative thinking or excessive perfectionism.

character traits, and in all three these persisted. Eight other patients were found to have compulsive character traits on second follow-up. It must be noted, however, that possibly they had these traits initially but they were not observed at that time. Therefore, the obsessive-compulsive phenomena either as symptoms or as character traits also tended to persist.

Eleven patients were found to have the hypochondriacal symptom pattern, four as a principal feature of the presenting illness and seven at a milder level of intensity. Four of the eleven patients still had this symptom pattern on second follow-up, but seven did not. In addition, eight patients who had not had this symptom initially were found to have it on second follow-up at mild levels of intensity. The implication is that there is somewhat more shift in the hypochondriacal symptom pattern than in the others.

Three patients had psychophysiologic symptom patterns on the initial interview, one with migraine, two with asthma. These persisted. On second follow-up, two additional patients reported asthma for the first time, and thirteen reported tension headaches without any previous history of this difficulty. It must be mentioned here that on second follow-up we specifically asked about this particular symptom (see Chapter 2), whereas we had not done so on initial evaluation.

To summarize: The conversion symptom pattern is striking in that it presents itself in a dramatic and intense manner and then disappears. Likewise, the phobic is dramatic in presentation but does not disappear and tends to persist at a subclinical level. The obsessive-compulsive phenomenon also persists. The hypochondriacal symptom pattern tends to show more shift, and the psychophysiologic both persists and increases.

Miscellaneous Signs on Examination

On examination, there were a number of miscellaneous signs which did not comprise any symptom pattern but were of interest (see Chapter 2). Concentration difficulty as tested by the Serial Seven Examination remained at about the same level (forty-seven on initial evaluation, forty on second follow-up). However, it varied by diagnosis, those with psychoneurosis showing a decrease from 75 per cent to 33 per cent, and those with schizophrenia and personality disorder showing little change. Obesity had a striking increase: ten on initial evaluation and twenty-one on first follow-up, and fully one-third of the patients on second follow-up were obese.

We close this section with two features usually associated with schizophrenia that we found to be equally associated with personality disorder. One is a behavioral expression of psychopathology: poor socialization; the other is a finding on examination: blunted affect. Poor socialization was found in twenty-six patients on initial evaluation: 55 per cent of those with schizophrenia, 30 per cent of those with personality disorder, and 25 per cent of those with psychoneurosis. On follow-up it was found in none of the patients with psychoneurosis, 22 per cent of those with schizophrenia, and 24 per cent of those with personality disorder. Twenty-eight patients had blunted affect on the initial evaluation: 66 per cent of those with schizophrenia, 16 per cent of those with psychoneurosis, and 33 per cent of those with personality disorder. Though it was more common among schizophrenics, it was certainly common enough among patients with personality disorders. On follow-up there were twenty-three with this finding: 28 per cent of those with schizophrenia, 25 per cent of those with psychoneurosis, and 36 per cent of those with personality disorder.

We can now recapitulate the findings in terms of the question to which this chapter was addressed. Some symptom patterns disappear, some increase in incidence, others diminish in intensity to a subclinical level, while still others show a remarkable degree of persistence. Although we cannot evaluate the effect of treatment on this persistence, or the possibility of symptom pattern shifts in the intervals between the interviews, we can say that at three different points in their lives (age sixteen, age eighteen, and age twenty-one) these patients showed remarkable persistence in many of their symptom patterns. Thus the findings at the symptom pattern level, particularly for patients with personality disorder, confirm the findings at the diagnostic level: The clinical picture of these adolescents as they progress through and emerge from adolescence not only tends toward clearer differentiation of diagnostic category but also shows persistence of many symptom patterns.

We cannot confirm the relationship of adolescent turmoil to instability of psychiatric symptomatology, but our evidence is supportive of another theory. It suggests that in those with personality disorder adolescent turmoil must be considered a factor secondary to that of the increasing demands of later adult life as a formative influence on the development and course of their psychiatric illness. The gradual termination of their adolescent years seems a trauma equal to, or greater perhaps than, adolescent turmoil. It forces them to leave the protected shores of childhood for the last time and tosses them like castaways, alone in a leaky boat, on the turbulent sea of adulthood. Many of the cracks and leaks, previously trifling by reason of the shallow waters of childhood, assume alarming proportions. Alone and unprepared to cope with the stresses of adult life, they quickly run afoul of their environment. Previously overprotective parents then frequently become annoyed and withdraw support, their dependency needs become increasingly frustrated, their weakened ego structures give way under the strain, and they require more and more symptomatology to maintain adjustment. Acting-out persists and hampers their efforts to cope, and depression as well as other symtoms, such as obesity and headaches, come to the fore.

CHAPTER 12

THEY DIDN'T GROW OUT OF IT

Who, in his tenderest years, finds some new lovely
thing, his hope is high and he flies on the wings of
his manhood: Better than riches are his thoughts—
man's pleasure is a short time growing and it falls
to the ground as quickly, when an unlucky twist of
thought loosens its roots.

—Pindar

ARE THESE ADOLESCENTS "just in a phase," and do they, as
current theory suggests, grow out of their difficulties? This theory
has such an unquestioned implicit acceptance by psychiatrists who
work with adolescents and is so deeply embedded in their thinking
that in case presentation after case presentation, regardless of the type
or intensity of the clinical picture, the opinion is proffered that the
patient "may grow out of his difficulties." It pervades the psychoanalytic literature in the expressed opinions of such authors as Josselyn [39], Erickson [22], Deutsch [19], Blos [16], Eissler [21], and
Anna Freud [26].

The effect of this theory when, as seems to be the case, it is applied
indiscriminately to the evaluation of all symptomatic adolescents is
obvious: It breeds a false security, a feeling that one can wait to start
treatment since it can be assumed that the patient's problems are due
to growth and will disappear with time. Such inaction, based on the
assumption that time is on the side of the patient, may actually do
him a disservice, for this study reveals that the truth of the matter
may often be the reverse. Many symptomatic adolescents are not
going to "grow out of their difficulties."

What does growing out of difficulties mean? We defined the general term *difficulties* to mean functional impairment. This concept,
traditionally made use of by the psychiatrist in his office, is defined in
the APA manual as "the degree to which a patient's total capacity to
function is impaired by his psychiatric illness." In terms of functional
impairment, then, growing out of difficulties means that the adolescent's symptoms subside enough to enable him to complete his
schooling and engage in satisfactory work and social activity.

Table 8 presents follow-up functional psychiatric impairment by diagnosis. We then discuss each level of impairment of function, citing case illustrations.

Table 8. Follow-up Functional Impairment by Diagnosis

Level of Impairment	Diagnosis						
		Personality Disorder					
	Schizophrenia (No.)	Sociopath (No.)	Passive-Aggressive (No.)	Miscellaneous (No.)	With Epilepsy (No.)	Character Neurosis (No.)	Total (No.)
Minimal	0	0	4	1	1	9	15
Mild	5	0	4	1	0	2	12
Moderate	6	3	9	2	2	0	22
Severe	7	7	3	4	2	0	23
Total	18	10	20	8	5	11	72

Observing the column on the extreme right, first we notice that forty-five, or 62 per cent, of the patients have moderate or severe impairment. Breaking this down by diagnosis, we see that those with character neurosis do well, all having only minimal or mild impairment of function, whereas those with schizophrenia and personality disorder do poorly, 75 per cent having moderate or severe impairment of function. When the personality disorders are subdivided by type, it becomes apparent that 100 per cent of the sociopaths, 63 per cent of those with a passive-aggressive disorder, 75 per cent of the miscellaneous, and 80 per cent of the epileptics continue to have moderate or severe impairment of function. Considering that on initial evaluation almost all of these patients were moderately or severely impaired, we can say that clearly, in terms of functional impairment, they did not grow out of their difficulties. Table 8 gives the bare bones of the story. To fill in the muscle and flesh let us consider in more detail the cases at each level of impairment.

Moderate and Severe Impairment

SCHIZOPHRENIA

Of the seven patients whose functional impairment is severe, six are in state hospitals and one is in prison. Two have been in the state hospital for five years, two for two years, and two for one year. The six moderately impaired, though able to stay out of a hospital, have been unable to maintain a consistently satisfactory adjustment at work or in their social life. The following case is an example.

A fifteen-and-a-half-year-old boy referred by the school gave a history of marked anxiety, tension, and poor performance in school which began early in life and was intensified at the age of thirteen and associated with his social life's decreasing to the point of his becoming an isolate. In addition, he rebelled passively against both mother and father. His school difficulties were so severe that he had to be placed in a special school. On examination, he was anxious, tense, and rebellious. He denied any problems but showed marked concentration difficulty, a severe thinking disorder, and a blunted and inappropriate affect.

When seen on follow-up five years later at the age of twenty-two, he had improved. After recurrent failures due to the concentration difficulty produced by his severe thinking disorder he had finally been graduated from high school at the age of twenty-two and had recently obtained a job as a shipping clerk. He planned to attend medical technician school. In the interim he had suffered from a duodenal ulcer and recurrent depressions. He was markedly dependent on his father and grandmother and had no social life, no interest in the opposite sex. He was fearful about driving cars and compulsive and perfectionistic, being quite meticulous about his room and belongings. On examination he appeared anxious and grossly immature. He showed a severe thinking disorder, flat affect, and suggestions of paranoid thinking coupled with a continued denial of any problems.

PERSONALITY DISORDER

The seven sociopaths who had had severe functional impairment at the age of sixteen, plus or minus, continued to show severe functional impairment on follow-up as judged by the following typical interim reports: inability to hold a job, drinking, gambling, taking drugs, police arrests, conflicts in relationships with people, and recurrent bouts of anxiety and depression, some with paranoid trends. The three passive-aggressives who had shown severe functional impairment still had a multitude of symptoms on follow-up, including anxiety, depression, psychoneurotic and psychophysiologic complaints, and bodily symptoms, besides marked inhibitions of emotional expression due to their passive-aggressive character structure (in school, at work, etc.). The ten moderately impaired passive-aggressives also suffered from anxiety, depression, and psychophysiologic complaints as well as difficulties with initiative. They were able to finish school in a checkered sort of fashion and to maintain themselves for varying periods at work, but usually at jobs well below their potential. Two case examples follow, the first showing severe impairment, the second moderate impairment.

A fifteen-and-a-half-year-old girl with a childhood history of having been a "feeding problem" and of soiling, had chronic feelings of inferiority, temper tantrums, nail-biting, thumb-sucking, and asthma. Since adolescence there had been recurrent episodes of depression and elation. She was repetitively a truant from school and in great conflict with her family. She came to the clinic in the setting of a depression, following rejection by a boy because she repulsed his sexual advances, and an impulsive suicide attempt by swallowing fifteen aspirin tablets and five sleeping pills. On examination, it was our opinion that the patient had no major affect or thinking disorder but that she represented a personality disorder, either inadequate or sociopathic in type.

The follow-up interview five and a half years later, when the patient was twenty-one, revealed that her interim course had been one of progressive deterioration. By age eighteen, she had attempted to attend college away from home but had become depressed, gained a lot of weight, felt rejected, and then returned home. At this time she engaged in sexual play with boys without excitement but was fearful of sexual intercourse. By age twenty-one, the patient had entirely given up school, had left home, and had lived alone for two months. She had started to use narcotics and had been picked up by the police for stealing. She had become involved in a sadomasochistic sexual relationship with an older man of unsavory character.

A fourteen-year-old boy, a psychopath, had complaints of anxiety, restlessness, concentration difficulty, school failures, obesity, rivalry with his sister, excessive concern about money, and conflict with an overprotective, overindulgent mother and a rejecting father.

When seen on follow-up six years later, at age twenty, he had been in college for two years but had failed several subjects. One failure was due to his inability to get up in the morning, which he later circumvented by arranging afternoon classes. On the rare occasions when he studied, he suffered from concentration difficulties, daydreaming, and procrastination. He was obese, impulsive and dependent, manipulative, and in conflict with his father. He was in constant need of money, which he spent impulsively whenever he had any. When examined on follow-up, both the patient and his mother denied the presence of problems. Being away at school had minimized the tension involved in the conflict with his father, and by getting a job he had managed to augment his income to better satisfy his need for money.

We have illustrated how forty-five adolescents, far from growing out of their difficulties, continued to show overt evidence of the persistence of symptomatology and both severe and moderate impairment of functioning as evidenced by continuing maladjustment in schoolwork, in interpersonal relations at home, and in their social life. Let us turn now to the twenty-seven with the best outcome, those minimally and mildly impaired.

Minimal and Mild Impairment

These twenty-seven, five with schizophrenia, eleven with personality disorder, and eleven with character neurosis, are able to function with minimal impairment; they go to school or have steady jobs, maintain a social life, and have some heterosexual relationship. Five patients who had been diagnosed as schizophrenic were found on follow-up to be able to carry on in the following occupations: secretary, photographer, television electrician, music teacher, and college student. Three live at home, one at college, another away from home. All function more or less on their own, in that they have some social life and some relationship with the opposite sex. Two had five years of treatment to attain a consistent level of adjustment, while two others attained it within six months of treatment and one had no treatment. However, in all five, adjustment appears tenuous and subject to reversal with future stress. There are many complaints of recurrent anxiety and depression, insomnia, tension, and headaches; one male patient expressed a concern about homosexuality. The following is a case illustration:

A fifteen-year-old boy, on initial examination, described his obsessive homicidal thoughts about his parents, overconcern with masturbation, borderline functioning in school for many years, and a state of social isolation. In the intervening period, with the aid of treatment, he had exhibited a slow, gradual improvement to the point of being, at the time of follow-up at age twenty, a sophomore in a technical college. He was able to live at school, coming home only for weekends. Although the intensity and frequency of his homicidal thoughts had diminished markedly, they were still present. He still had some difficulty in school as well as headaches, insomnia, recurrent mild depression, and recurrent concern about homosexuality. He remained dependent on his mother and had had considerable anxiety about aggressive impulses. He had just started to date and consequently had never been emotionally or sexually involved with a girl. He appeared immature on examination and was socially aloof and withdrawn. Though clearly functioning better than on the initial interview five years previously, he continued to have symptoms and his functioning, though rated as only mildly impaired, was considerably short of an optimal level of adjustment.

Turning to the eleven patients diagnosed as having personality disorder, most of whom are of the subtype passive-aggressive, we find that, though their functioning has improved, they also show overt symptoms. All but one finished high school, commonly requiring extra time to do so; two are in college, two women work as secretaries, two are in the armed services, and five men work at miscellaneous jobs. They complain of recurrent anxiety and depression, headaches, insomnia, feelings of inadequacy, obesity, dysmenorrhea, and overconcern with other bodily feelings and functions. The following is an illustrative case:

A sixteen-year-old boy, with a passive-aggressive personality disorder, when first seen was markedly depressed, failing in school, hostile toward and in open conflict with a cold and distant father, and in social difficulty with his peers, as he had been since childhood. He did not graduate from high school, left home at age eighteen and "for lack of anything else to do" went into the army, where he experienced a dramatic change upon joining the Baptist Church at age nineteen. He had a good relationship with the minister and changed from being passive and withdrawn to being active socially and intensely interested in the Baptist Church and religion, to the point of evangelizing. He disliked his army work, hated authority figures, and exhibited strong sadistic trends in his humor. Though he dated girls, he avoided emotional commitment and had no heterosexual activity. In addition, he had withdrawn from both mother and father. He admitted to anxiety, insomnia, and feelings of inadequacy and on examination showed severe repression, reaction formation, intellectualization, and denial.

Lastly, we find that the eleven with character neurosis, eight of whom are women, function at a higher level than those in the other two diagnostic groups. All finished high school with little difficulty. They attained better grades in school, have more interests and activities and more goal direction in their lives, and are more actively involved with the opposite sex. Four women have married and are successful housewives with children, two are in college, and two work as secretaries. One of the three men is in college, another in Marine officer candidate school, and a last works steadily at a job, which is more in keeping with his education and intellectual endowment. However, they have recurrent anxiety and depression and mild phobic and psychophysiologic complaints. Following is a case example:

A seventeen-year-old girl, with a mixed character neurosis with anxiety and hysterical and depressive features, on initial examination gave a history since age fourteen of intense anxiety attacks before each date, manifested by restlessness, chills, vomiting, and anorexia; recurrent spells of depression with suicidal preoccupation; and one suicidal attempt with aspirin. There was also marked conflict with both parents, whom the patient saw as critical and complaining, and rivalry with her nine-year-old sister. Menarche occurred at age eleven with a weight gain of 17 pounds, but there was a past history of vomiting when "excited" from age five to age eleven. Her school and social history were good.

When seen at age twenty-two, the patient had been married for three years, had one child, and functioned well as a housewife with outside interests and activities. Nevertheless, this adjustment was a costly one, with recurrent episodes of both anxiety and depression. These occur particularly in the setting of rivalry with her mother-in-law for her husband, upon whom she is excessively dependent. She represses her anger at her mother-in-law's apparent attempts to win more affection from her husband and thereupon she develops depression and insomnia. In addition to being dependent on her husband, she appears compliant, passive, and immature and reports perverse fantasies in order to enjoy sexual activity. Her conflict with her own mother had disappeared but she has remained aloof from her father.

To summarize: Despite the fact that they function well, all twenty-seven patients continue to reveal some such symptomatology as just described, which more or less seriously interferes with an ideal adjustment consonant with a "maturity" appropriate for their age.

A more fundamental and more complex question is raised about the whole group of twenty-seven patients who have done well. Defining difficulties in terms of functioning, we found that approximately two-thirds of the adolescent patients do not grow out of their difficulties, while approximately one-third do. This definition, though adequate for most purposes, as we know from psychoanalysis, leaves something to be desired, since often patients such as obsessive-compulsives do learn to function well—but at the cost of, rather than through the expression of, their inner emotional needs. We would, therefore, like to know more about these patients. If we now define difficulties, not in terms of functioning, but in terms of underlying conflicts with regard to dependency needs and to sexual and aggressive impulses, we want to know to what extent the patients have made some comfortable resolution of conflicts in these three key areas. We want to know also to what extent, in the course of this process of resolution, their character structure had remained free from psychopathologic traits, thereby enabling the diverse elements of their mental apparatus to blend harmoniously to produce self-actualization or optimal functioning. Unfortunately our study was not designed to elicit these data, since it is based on three interviews only with patient and mother over a five-year period. Nevertheless, it would be shortsighted indeed not to utilize the material we do have to make what contribution we can, keeping in mind that it is at best impressionistic. From this point of view we again reviewed the twenty-seven patients minimally impaired, assuming that in the others the presence of more than mild impairment was evidence of the fact that they had been unable to resolve their conflicts.

SCHIZOPHRENIA

Though three patients have managed to gain some measure of independence, all five continue to show dependency on and conflict with the mother.

As to sexual adjustment: Two male patients have dated rarely and have had no emotional or sexual involvement with girls. A twenty-one-year-old girl puts off the marriage proposals of her boy friend, with whom she nevertheless has regular sexual intercourse but to whom she cannot commit herself wholeheartedly. A boy of twenty six months ago broke up with a girl upon whom he was emotionally dependent; they had engaged in petting without sexual intercourse, because he said the sexual intercourse he had had four years before had made him "feel rotten after." Another young man, age twenty, has been going steady with a girl for six months, but he is unwilling to divulge any further sexual information.

Aggressive impulses continue to be a source of anxiety and are handled by such defense mechanisms as suppression, repression, projection, or withdrawal. The character structure of these five patients seems marked by traits of immaturity, suspiciousness, social aloofness, and trouble with self-organization. The case illustration on pages 123–124 demonstrates that these patients still have difficulties with dependency needs and sexual aggressive impulses.

PERSONALITY DISORDER

In seven patients, there is clear evidence of dependency on and conflict with the mother that has lessened very little over the course of time. This is handled either by their continuing to live at home, which may enable them to function better than they otherwise would, or by withdrawal from the parents as well as the home. In those who remain at home, the conflict with the mother seems to persist almost intact and unabated from early adolescence. For example, two girls, both twenty-one, are both obese and living at home. One shows passive rebellion toward, and withdrawal from, her mother, and the other has episodes of depression.

As to sexual adjustment, two others have had sexual intercourse. One, a girl twenty-one, later declined a marriage proposal; the other, a boy twenty-two, has not allowed himself to become emotionally committed to a girl. Five have been emotionally involved to the point of going steady, and five have dated without ever going steady or having sexual intercourse.

Aggression continues to present a problem, which is handled by such defenses as repression, reaction-formation and intellectualization, rebellious acting-out, or passively by provocation and withdrawal. Almost all give evidence of some pathologic character traits; frequently they vary from being passive, submissive, overcompliant, lacking initiative, with other immature emotional expression, to being withdrawn, suspicious, and perfectionistic, with much repression and denial of emotion.

The case description on page 124 provides a most illustrative example of reaction-formations to aggressive and sexual impulses. This patient evidently transferred his dependency needs to the Baptist minister and, through identification with him and the church, changed from exhibiting a passive to exhibiting an active response to his environment, being highly motivated by his new religious standards. Although he functioned better, it was at the cost of, rather than a satisfactory resolution of, his aggressive and sexual impulses, and he developed a markedly rigid, defensive character structure. The influence is justified in that his elaborate reaction-formations have left him potentially vulnerable to future stress.

CHARACTER NEUROSIS

Seven of the eleven patients in this category show evidence of a continued dependency on the mother, which, however, lessened in intensity and seems to have a less pervasive effect on their functioning than was found in those with personality disorder. For example, a boy who used to be overwhelmed by his mother's nagging is now freer to act on his own initiative and is more self-assertive. Six patients are able to live away from home. In contrast to those with personality disorder, only two patients have had neither intercourse nor a close emotional relationship with someone of the opposite sex. Two of the four married women describe sexual difficulties. Of the remaining seven, four are girls, three of whom have gone steady for at least two years, indulging in petting but no sexual intercourse. Four patients gave no evidence of difficulties in managing aggression, but the rest exhibit prominent defenses of repression and reaction-formation. Pathologic character traits, found in almost all, consist of rigidity, perfectionism, and compulsiveness, with less immaturity than was characteristic of those with schizophrenia and personality disorder.

If we once again study the case illustration on page 125, we may infer that the patient transferred her dependency needs from the mother to the husband, and that she continues to have conflict over sexual and aggressive impulses, as well as a character structure which shows such traits as rigid perfectionism, overcompliance, and passivity, plus evidences of immaturity.

The findings suggest that those who appear to grow out of their difficulties on a functional level nevertheless continue to show conflict with regard to dependency needs and sexual and aggressive impulses. They also have some frankly pathologic character traits. Rather than resolving their conflicts in the areas of dependency, sex, and aggression, they seem to have found ways to deal with them that have enabled them to function better. It cannot be denied, however, that the persistence of these conflicts makes them vulnerable to a variety of environmental stresses while at the same time the pathologic character traits impair their flexibility to respond to stress. That is, rather than growing out of their difficulties, they have found ways to adjust to them, which, while allowing them to function better, leaves them vulnerable to future stress.

Let us return to the starting point of this chapter to see what bearing these results have on current theory. Clearly the truth of the matter, at least in this group, is the reverse of current theory. Time was not on the side of the patients; they did not grow out of their difficulties. By far the majority, particularly those with schizophrenia and personality disorder, were not able to make even a functional adjustment but continued to show both symptoms and impairment of functioning. A smaller number of those with schizophrenia and personality disorder, and all of those with character neurosis, though they managed to make a functional adjustment to their difficulties, did so by finding better ways to deal with their conflicts rather than by resolving them, and consequently remain vulnerable to future stress.

In attempting to generalize from these results, we must advance a few reservations. Although this study like all studies has its methodological handicaps, it is the only systematic attempt to test current theory against actual clinical material. The evidence is strongest at the level of functional impairment. The evidence for failure to resolve conflicts and the persistence of pathologic character traits, while impressionistic, is still persuasive. The small number of patients raises an important question. Do we have a group who are unusually sick? Since our admission policies are the same as most outpatient clinics, these patients are fairly representative of a clinic population. They were selected as the "least sick" of 300 who applied for admission, and they do not vary greatly from those we see in private practice and, I would venture to guess, from those seen by most psychiatrists not working with schools. Nevertheless, it would be helpful to have similar studies of other clinic populations. A more likely possibility is that these patients are actually sicker than those seen in other settings such as a prep school or college where a psychiatrist is more readily available to consult for milder, more acute difficulties. However, keeping these reservations in mind it seems reasonable to conclude that the theory as at present conceived is not applicable to many patients, particularly those with schizophrenia and personality disorder and even some with neurosis, in whom adolescent turmoil is an incidental rather than a decisive influence. The implication is that the psychiatric significance of adolescent turmoil has been overestimated.

Psychotherapy

How does psychiatric treatment affect the clinical outcome? Did the patients fail to overcome their difficulties because they did not receive psychotherapy? Was the psychotherapy inadequate? Or did they show some improvement with psychotherapy that was primarily symptomatic? We have the same problem here as we did with the study of underlying conflicts: This study was not designed to evaluate psychiatric treatment. However, again as was the case with underlying conflicts, we do have some information which, while not part of the research project itself, may cast some light on the question of the effect of treatment. Forty-two patients received psychotherapy, thirty at the Payne Whitney Clinic. We reviewed the entire treatment record, in some cases of three or four years' duration, to answer three questions. Did the patient improve under psychiatric treatment? If so, how did psychiatric treatment help? If psychiatric treatment did not help, why not?

SCHIZOPHRENIA

Of the five patients with the best outcome, four were treated and one was not. The last patient was a sixteen-year-old boy (see the case history under Adjustment Reaction of Adolescence, in Chapter 5) with a history from age twelve of social withdrawal, anxiety, concentration difficulty, and school failures. At age fifteen and a half he had an acute onset of the delusion that people thought that circles under his eyes indicated masturbation. Without treatment his delusions disappeared, he was able to graduate from high school, and he is now working as a television technician and has recently established his own independent living away from home. One could possibly infer from this case that the acute upheaval of early adolescence precipitated the patient's delusions and that as he grew older and the turmoil subsided he made some adjustment to these impulses so that the acute delusion disappeared without treatment.

The other four patients seemed to be helped by psychiatric treatment. One, a severely disorganized schizophrenic, saw the same doctor once a week for four years, during which time he was hospitalized for seven months. He showed remarkable improvement and at twenty-two, graduated from college, was pursuing a career as a music teacher. The other three patients, treated from one to three years, all improved in a setting of a good relationship with their therapist, to whom they spoke freely, mostly about current problems and activities. There was no evidence, however, that underlying conflicts were dealt with.

This optimistic picture of improvement with psychiatric treatment seems to be contradicted by those who were moderately impaired on follow-up. All six patients received an average of two and a half years of outpatient therapy. One, treated at Payne Whitney, seen once a week, had a good relationship with the therapist, talked freely about underlying conflicts as well as current activities, and showed definite improvement over the course of the year of treatment, as did her mother. Within a short time after treatment, however, the patient relapsed. The data on the other five patients were insufficient to permit any impression. The contradiction continues when we study the seven patients severely impaired at the time of follow-up. They received a number of kinds of treatment, varying from one year outpatient to six years in a state hospital. One seen at Payne Whitney Clinic for six months seemed to develop a negative transference toward his therapist.

Thus those with a good outcome improved with psychiatric treatment, apparently because of a good relationship with the therapist, with whom they could discuss current feelings and activities, and without any deeper therapy. It is harder to interpret the effect of psychiatric treatment on those who did not do so well. Although they had a great deal of psychiatric treatment, they are still doing poorly, but the possibility remains that they might have done even worse without treatment. The findings cause one to reflect again on how central the severity of the patient's illness must be. One patient with an acute onset, with a sexual delusion, does well without treatment. A number responded well to treatment, but an even larger number with a great deal of treatment continue to have great difficulty.

CHARACTER NEUROSIS

There is an equally contradictory picture when we study the effect of treatment on those with character neurosis. Four patients received no treatment, three stopped treatment after a few interviews, and four were treated from one to three years. However, the outcomes of all eleven are similar. Of the three patients who stopped treatment, two did so after six to eight interviews, because of either lack of motivation or intense or improperly handled resistance. One patient became suicidal under treatment, and, when hospitalization was advised, he refused and stopped treatment. Nevertheless, this did not prevent him from having a good outcome. The four patients who were treated improved in the setting of a good relationship with the therapist, with whom they ventilated their feelings about current situations and activities. In none of the four is there evidence that prominent underlying conflicts were picked up and dealt with by the therapist. For example, one patient spoke frankly about social inadequacies, perfectionism, and the need to do better in school, while problems with dependency, sex, and aggression were not mentioned. But they did improve, even though these themes were not discussed. In each of these four cases the mother also improved; she became more realistic about setting limits, less oversolicitous, or more interested and affectionate toward her child.

Since all those with character neurosis did well, it is difficult to come to any conclusions. On the surface, it did not seem to matter whether treatment was absent, was stopped after a few interviews, or was prolonged. In considering the findings we must not overlook the possibility that there are finer differences in outcome among these patients that we did not discern. In addition, those untreated might have done better with treatment, and those with treatment might not have done so well without it. We begin to see in those with character neurosis who were treated a possibility that will be developed further with the personality disorder group: The fact that the patients who were treated function well but have not resolved dependency, aggressive, and sexual conflicts may reflect an inadequate consideration of these conflicts in their treatment.

PERSONALITY DISORDER

Seventeen patients received psychiatric treatment, six for six months, six for about a year, one for three years, and four for only a few interviews. Seven improved, six were unimproved, and four stopped treatment. The effect of psychiatric treatment on outcome is suggested by the fact that on follow-up five of the seven patients who improved under treatment were moderately impaired and two mildly impaired. In other words, though they improved under treatment, when seen later they were still having considerable trouble. The prominent theme in the treatment of those who improved is that of an individual who readily established a dependent relationship, had presenting complaints of anxiety, depression, and environmental conflicts, and ventilated his feelings readily about current activities and problems. In the course of treatment, the anxiety and depression subsided, the environmental conflicts became minimized, and the patient's functioning improved. However, such basic characterologic problems as passivity, dependency, immaturity, and negativism were inadequately dealt with, so that although the patient did improve, when he left treatment he ran into further problems, best indicated by the fact that five of the seven who improved were on follow-up still considered to be moderately impaired. The following is an example:

A thirteen-year-old boy presented a history since age ten, when his father died, of intense conflict with his mother and brother, excessive lying, stealing, truancy, and failing in school. The patient was seen in treatment for about a year. He had a dependent relationship with his therapist, and his interviews consisted mostly of discussions of current activities and airing of a long series of complaints about the mother's rejection and nagging behavior, his anger and counterprovocations, and his need to assert his masculinity. The therapist supported the patient's constructive activity and tried to redirect his anger. The mother's interviews consisted of repetitive, hostile, and rejecting complaints about the patient which yielded little to therapeutic intervention. In the course of treatment, however, the mother's rejecting behavior was somewhat modified, and the patient's school functioning and behavior at home also improved.

When we saw the patient again, at eighteen, he had left high school, where he was failing in two subjects, and was working in a supermarket. He complained of migraine headaches and reported that the conflict with the mother was still present, but decreased in intensity, the patient tending to withdraw and rebel passively. Rivalry with the brother continued as before. The patient's hostility was easily aroused and he frequently blew up at his job and then also suffered recurrent depressions. He spent a great deal of time sleeping and had withdrawn from his usual social life.

Eleven of the patients with personality disorder, ten of them moderately or severely impaired on follow-up, either did not improve with treatment or stopped treatment after a few sessions. In those who did not respond, there were a number of themes: In several cases the therapist, threatened by the patient's acting-out behavior, responded either without firmness or punitively, thereby repeating the patient's problems with the parents. In others, despite the therapist's efforts, it was not possible to circumvent the patient's resistance. In still others the patient's basic character problems were not effectively dealt with as part of the treatment.

A seventeen-year-old girl, treated for one year, established a dependent relationship with her therapist, spoke freely of her need for her mother's love, of anger at the mother's hostile rejection, of acting-out her anger to provoke the mother, and of seeking satisfaction of her needs through dependent relationships with boys. She spoke too of being afraid of sexual feelings and therefore of dating homosexual boys. The mother, however, in treatment was so rejecting of the patient and so narcissistic and preoccupied with her own conflicts with her husband that it was not possible to make much progress in changing her attitudes toward the daughter. Nevertheless, the patient's depression improved by the end of the year. Although she readily verbalized her hostility over the frustration of her dependency needs and the acting-out of this hostility, apparently no effort was made to help the patient gain control or to define alternate ways of dealing with these feelings. When seen later, at twenty-four, the patient showed continued difficulty with control of these impulses.

In summary: Sixteen of the thirty patients treated improved—five with schizophrenia, four with character neurosis, and seven with personality disorder. In most cases the improvement seemed to consist of the alleviation of presenting symptoms and complaints in the setting of a dependent relationship with the therapist. The fact that the fundamental underlying conflicts and the basic defects in character structure were effectively dealt with in so few cases may have something to do with our finding that even those who function well five years later continue to have these conflicts and pathologic character traits. It also suggests that we should be extremely cautious about judging the enduring nature of what for the most part seems to be symptomatic improvement.

SECTION V

ANOTHER FACET OF ADOLESCENT TURMOIL

CHAPTER 13

COMPARING PATIENTS WITH CONTROLS

> There are many persons who appear to be in good health, and whom only a physician will discern at first sight not to be in good health.
>
> —Plato: *Gorgias*, 494

T HE FOREGOING TWELVE CHAPTERS, dealing with the relationship of adolescent turmoil to those who are psychiatrically ill, cover three of the four elements of current theory as presented in Chapter 1. Chapters 13 and 14 will deal with the last element of the theory—the concept that adolescent turmoil causes psychiatric symptoms to be common and transient in most adolescents. This concept, developed primarily through the study of patients alone, beclouds the evaluation of the symptomatic adolescent by implying that the differences between patients and nonpatients are small. It must be tested against a community sample of adolescents who have not consulted a psychiatrist. Would they, as theory suggests, show symptomatology comparable to that seen in patients?

To put the matter to a practical test, our patient group was compared with a control group of 101 adolescents. This chapter describes how the control group was selected and examined then compares the symptomatology and functioning of the two groups. (Details of coding and analysis of the data can be found in the Appendix.)

Systematic Method

SELECTION OF A CONTROL GROUP

The control group consisted of 101 adolescents from the community who had never been seen for consultation or treatment by a psychologist, psychiatrist, or social worker. To minimize the possibility that any differences between the two groups could be due to demographic characteristics, we matched the controls to the patients for age, grade,

137

sex, race, religion, and type of school attended. We decided against a control group of "normal adolescents," since it required a prior definition of "normality" which we wanted to emerge from the findings. We also decided against a "symptom-free" group, since one of the central questions in adolescent psychiatry is how much symptomatology is "normally" present in adolescence. Although all matching adolescents who agreed to participate in the study were interviewed, those who were found to have had a prior consultation were excluded from the final group of 101.

RANDOM SAMPLING AT THE SCHOOLS

We selected the controls by random sampling techniques from twenty-seven of the sixty-six schools attended by the patients, since many were similar in educational level, subject focus, sponsorship, location, size, and type of student body. The location of the school was used in a general way to control for socioeconomic differences.

We made every effort to get in touch with a family by telephone or mail before we discarded a name from the random list, eventually getting our sample of 101 adolescents from over 650 families. It was necessary to consult the family to match for race and religion because the school records did not contain this information. We explained the study first to the parents and then to the adolescent, obtaining the consent of both for participation. Parental permission was also obtained in writing, a copy being given to the school. We located 172 adolescents who met all the criteria; of this number, 42 or 24 per cent, refused to take part in the study, 17 were eliminated because of a history of prior consultation, and 12 were excluded because of matching errors.

An approach was needed which would allow the examiners to elicit psychiatric information from adolescents who came without presenting complaints or even preparation to discuss their personal life experiences. Interviews, held at the school, were partially structured so as to bring up areas of conflict by asking such open-ended questions as: "What problems do you think someone your age might have?" Both boys and girls focused on the *present*, with dating, friends, money, grades, and parents mentioned most frequently. When the *future* was mentioned, college and careers were seen as problematical.

Interviewed separately by two psychiatrists, the adolescents were seen by each for an hour. The first psychiatrist was guided by a schedule which covered the standard examination, along with school and social, personal, and family history. The second psychiatrist used a questionnaire devised after the initial patient interviews to investigate a broad spectrum of symptomatology and to pick up, we hoped, any symptoms missed during the less-structured first interview. Almost all parents were visited in their homes by a social worker, often during the evening. The schedule used during the two-hour parental interview was similar to the usual clinical examination. After each interview the examiners wrote a summary of their findings.

SYMPTOM PATTERNS

Table 9 compares the symptom patterns of controls with patients.

Table 9.   Symptom Patterns: Controls Versus Patients

Symptom Pattern	Controls (N=101)	Patients (N=101)
Anxiety	65	73
Depression	41	35
Immature	15	18
Schizophrenic	6	22
Acting-out	19	48
Sexual difficulty	11	31
Hypochondriacal	3	14
Hysterical personality disorder	–	10
Conversion	–	9
Psychophysiologic	1	7
Organic reaction	–	1
Obsessive-compulsive	19	5
Phobic	11	7
Compulsive personality disorder	9	3
Total	200	283
Average number of symptoms	1.98	2.80
Absence of symptom patterns	17	4

We note first an average of 1.98 symptoms for the controls and 2.80 for the patients, which supports current theory that psychiatric symptoms are common in adolescents. Next, looking at the symptom patterns themselves, we see that the findings for the first three again support current theory. That is, anxiety, depression, and immature personality are fairly similar in the two groups; a substantial portion of both have anxiety and depression, with fewer showing immature personality. The next three symptom patterns show differences in the two groups which qualify current theory; i.e., schizophrenic, acting-out, and sexual difficulty are more common in the patients than in controls. Further differences are indicated by the next five symptom patterns—hypochondriacal, hysterical personality disorder, conversion, psychophysiologic, and organic reaction—which, while present in patients, were absent in or limited to few of the controls. The last three symptom patterns, obsessive-compulsive, phobic, and compulsive personality disorder, were more common in the controls than in the patients. On checking the coding we found that, unlike the rest of the symptom patterns, these last three were coded from the questionnaire rather than the clinical examination. We felt that the questionnaire, which was not used for the initial patient interviews, increased the number of symptom patterns detected and therefore the differences in these symptom patterns were probably a result of the difference in method. It is quite possible that a larger number of symptoms would have accrued to the patient group had the questionnaire been used for them.

Examining the depression and acting-out symptom patterns in more detail, we found additional differences. Although the symptom pattern of depression (see Appendix, Table 16) was equally common in both groups, there were fewer in the controls with severe depression as illustrated by the fact that only two had had suicidal thoughts and none had attempted suicide, whereas twelve of the patients had had suicidal thoughts and five had attempted suicide. This trend was elaborated in the acting-out symptom pattern, where differences between the two groups varied from antisocial behavior, which was equally common (four controls, five patients) though small in number, to rebellious behavior at school, which was moderately more common in the patients (eleven controls, eighteen patients), to stealing (two controls, ten patients) and sexual acting-out (one control, nine patients), which were much more common in patients than controls.

To further define the differences between the groups the two psychiatrists reviewed the symptom patterns for each adolescent and chose one as the principal symptom pattern (see Appendix, Table 16). Though not a clinical diagnosis, the principal symptom pattern is derived from the most outstanding symptom pattern for each subject. Table 10 presents the principal symptom patterns.

Table 10.   Principal Symptom Patterns: Controls Versus Patients

Principal Symptom Pattern	Controls (N=101)	Patients (N=101)
Anxiety	38	26
Depression	16	7
Acting-out	5	17
Schizophrenic	4	16
Immature	4	2
Sexual difficulty	1	4
Hypochondriacal	—	4
Hysterical personality disorder	—	6
Conversion	—	3
Psychophysiologic	—	2
Organic reaction	—	1
Obsessive-compulsive	5	3
Phobic	—	2
Compulsive personality disorder	1	—
Undesignated*	10	4
Absence of symptom patterns	17	4

* Refers to the presence of one or more symptom patterns, but one pattern did not predominate over another.

Anxiety, depression, and absence of a principal symptom pattern now characterize 70 per cent of the controls and only 37 per cent of the patients. On the other hand, schizophrenic and acting-out are present in 33 per cent of the patients and only 9 per cent of the controls. Moreover, the patients are distributed throughout all the principal symptom categories, except compulsive personality disorder, while the distribution of the controls is more limited.

To give further meaning to the principal symptom patterns we rated their intensity. The rating had four levels—absent, mild, moderate, and severe—and was based on definitions of the principal symptom patterns (see Appendix, Table 16). This rating was independent of other differences and was based on principal symptom pattern alone. Table 11 compares the symptom intensity rating for the controls and patients.

The controls are equally divided between absent-mild and moderate-

Table 11.   Symptom Intensity Rating: Controls Versus Patients

Symptom Intensity Rating	Controls (N=101)	Patients (N=101)
Absent	17	4
Mild	32	27
Moderate*	45	36
Severe	7	34

* Four of the patients who had not been assigned a rating of symptom intensity were placed in the moderate group based on the patient group's average.

severe symptom intensity, while the patients show one-third in the absent-mild group and two-thirds in the moderate-severe group. The greatest difference is seen at the severe level, which is five times greater for the patients than for the controls. The finding of moderate-severe symptom intensity in fifty-two controls supports current theory. However, further analysis of these fifty-two showed that 40 per cent had principal symptom patterns of anxiety and 20 per cent depression, with two having a principal symptom pattern of schizophrenia and four with acting-out. In other words, the moderate-severe symptom tended to be mostly anxiety and some depression rather than schizophrenia or acting-out.

This finding, based on descriptive rather than diagnostic criteria, raises an issue that will be pursued in later diagnostic studies, namely, that moderate-severe anxiety and depression may actually occur so commonly in both patients and community adolescents that they do not help to differentiate the former from the latter.

IMPAIRMENT OF FUNCTIONING

Table 12 compares the impairment of functioning of the two groups, academically and socially.* Observing first the average school impairment, we notice that the controls are one-half as impaired as the patients. As for distribution, the two groups have approximately the same number in the mild and moderate categories, the largest difference appearing in the severe category, which contains none of the controls and one-fourth of the patients.

Turning now to the social impairment, and again consulting the average first, we see that both groups are less impaired socially than

* See Appendix, Tables 18 and 19, for definitions.

Table 12.   Impairment of Functioning*

	School		Social	
Impairment	Controls (N=101)	Patients (N=101)	Controls (N=101)	Patients (N=101)
Minimal	53	32	67	49
Mild	28	26	15	18
Moderate	20	19	12	12
Severe	—	24	6	14
Unknown	—	—	1	8
Average impairment	.67	1.35	.57	.90

* The impairments were assigned the following scores: Minimal = 0, Mild = 1, Moderate = 2, Severe = 3. The average impairment for the group was assigned to the "unknowns" to obtain the overall average.

they were scholastically, and although the patients are more impaired socially than the controls, the difference is not so striking as was found for school impairment. The distribution repeats the pattern noted for school functioning in that a similar number of controls and patients are in the mild to moderate categories, with the largest difference in the severe category.

Twenty-one adolescents in the control group and nearly twice as many, thirty-eight, in the patient group showed both school and social impairment.

Before interpreting these findings let us mention a few of the methodologic limitations. Though our material, derived from a single series of interviews, limits our understanding of psychodynamics, we believe we obtained an accurate clinical picture illustrative of the findings of the usual psychiatric consultation. The results at this point are based on systematic, descriptive data to help control the comparison of the same item in two different groups. Later, after completion of the follow-up, when it is to be hoped that many of the controls will have completed their patterns of development, we intend to review the entire body of material from the clinical point of view.

According to the current theory that adolescent turmoil commonly produces psychiatric illness and symptomatology, we might have anticipated small differences between the two groups. Our findings support one aspect of the theory and qualify another. Although psychiatric symptoms were common among adolescents who had never seen a psychiatrist, their incidence was in the order of two for a control to three for a patient. However, the symptoms in controls tended to be primarily those of anxiety, depression, and immaturity and not the more psychiatrically serious symptoms of schizophrenia and personality disorder such as occurred in the patient group. In addition, the community adolescents functioned almost twice as well as the patients.

The Impact of Adolescent Turmoil

Now we must question whether these differences might be due to the fact that we have two special groups—one that is unusually "sick" and one that is uncommonly "well." The patients were selected as the "least sick" of 300 who applied for admission to the clinic, and they differed only slightly from those I see in my private practice. There are no other similar studies of community adolescents, but the levels of symptomatology reported for our controls do not differ much from those reported for adults in recent community prevalence studies [41, 74]. Thus our two groups are not "special." Granting that much of the current difficulty in conceptualizing the adolescent problem may have arisen from uncautious and too hasty generalizations, our findings do suggest the tentative hypothesis that the psychiatric significance of adolescent turmoil has been overestimated and that, except possibly in the areas of anxiety and depression, its psychiatric effects are not so ubiquitous as to make the symptomatology in community adolescents comparable to that seen in patients.

We anticipated that the 101 community adolescents, though they had never seen a psychiatrist, would provide a spectrum ranging from the healthy to the psychiatrically ill. The presence of schizophrenic symptomatology in six (see Table 9) of these adolescents, the number with moderate-severe anxiety and depression, and the twenty-one impaired both academically and socially support the view that a number are psychiatrically ill. Similarly, we expected the patients, though they came for consultation, to include a few who were not actually psychiatrically ill. Therefore, Chapter 14 gets closer to the essence of the difference between the two groups by comparing, not patients with controls, but the psychiatrically healthy with the psychiatrically ill.

CHAPTER 14

COMPARING THE RELATIVELY HEALTHY WITH THE PSYCHIATRICALLY ILL

> Look to your health; and if you have it, praise God, and value it next to a good conscience; for health is the second blessing that we mortals are capable of,— a blessing that money cannot buy.
> —Izaak Walton: *The Compleat Angler*

I T I S A P P R O P R I A T E to pose two questions: first, could a psychiatrist, using the traditional psychiatric concept of illness, select a group of healthy and a group of ill adolescents from these two patient and control groups? Second, if he could, would the differences between healthy and ill be greater than those already found between patients and controls? This chapter describes the characteristics of the relatively healthy and shows how they differ from the psychiatrically ill in symptoms, functioning, and family relationships.

By careful clinical review of all the material available for the 101 controls and for the 101 patients (see Chapter 2), we selected two groups: one that we could say with greatest confidence was relatively healthy and one that we could say with greatest confidence was ill. Using the traditional psychiatric criteria of symptoms and impairment of functioning, we defined as relatively healthy those adolescents who did not show significant symptomatology or impairment of functioning but who had a reasonable—not necessarily an optimal— state of functioning; and we defined as relatively ill those adolescents who had clear evidence of psychiatric symptomatology and impairment of functioning. We reserved a category of doubtful for individuals about whose status we were not certain.

Psychiatrically Ill

On clinical review we eliminated eight patients. In three the psychiatric status was doubtful, and in five the consultation seemed to

145

be a result of family conflict. All the latter five showed, as prominent features, conflict with a pressuring mother, a chief presenting symptom of anxiety, and some difficulty in school. This left ninety-three whom we confidently considered psychiatrically ill, an impression which was confirmed through follow-up five years later in seventy-two of the ninety-three.

Relatively Healthy

On clinical review of the control adolescents we found forty-one healthy and twenty-seven ill. We considered thirty-three doubtful; in twenty-four the doubt was whether they were healthy and in nine whether they were ill. Many of the twenty-four were excluded because we wanted a rigorous definition of the relatively healthy, and a broader definition might have included these subjects. Although they will be reported in detail in another publication, we illustrate below some of the types excluded:

1. One group showed characterologic features that hinted at, but did not establish, pathology, such as schizoid trends, immaturity, passivity, or obsessive-compulsive behavior.
2. Another group showed symptomatology that was clinically borderline, such as moderate anxiety, mild depression, episodes of gastrointestinal upsets, dysmenorrhea, or mild phobic features.
3. A final group showed moderate anxiety, occasional school failures, and conflict with parents.

We describe the composite present and past symptomatology of the relatively healthy, as noted on clinical review, along with one case example.

PRESENT SYMPTOMATOLOGY

Present symptoms tended to be single rather than multiple, of mild intensity, and episodic in duration: (1) anxiety, (2) depression, (3) compulsive traits (hand washing, avoiding cracks in the pavement, grouping letters into three's, bathing twice daily, hand clenching), (4) phobic traits (fear of heights, being alone, spiders, being hit by cars), (5) somatic complaints (headaches, backaches, gastrointestinal upsets, dysmenorrhea), (6) character traits (oversensitivity, detachment in relationships, rigid intellectualization, perfectionism).

PAST SYMPTOMATOLOGY

The evidence of past symptomatology is less adequate than that for the present, since parents were occasionally uncooperative in the interview, showed denial themselves, or could not remember: (1) separation anxiety, six (one kept the bottle until age three, another got up nightly until age six to see if mother was there, a third was afraid to stay alone, two had anxiety in going to kindergarten and had to leave, and another had difficulty in giving up the blanket and bottle); (2) somatic complaints (episodic histories of abdominal pain without vomiting, four; headaches, three; dysmenorrhea, one); (3) psychoneurotic symptoms (teeth grinding, one; fear of needles, one); (4) other symptoms (allergies, two; poor eating, three; enuresis, three—one to age four, one to age eleven, and one to age five; stuttering, three—one to a few months, one to age nine; obesity, two; speech difficulty, one; overcompliance, two; poor social life, two).

EXAMPLE OF A RELATIVELY HEALTHY PERSON

A. C., the second of three children, is an attractive brown-eyed sixteen-year-old girl, in her junior year in high school. Intelligent, outgoing, and popular, she is an "A" student, interested in music, playing both piano and violin, active in sports, and involved in a plethora of social activities. She dates about once a week, has never gone steady, and wonders about meeting the right man and getting married. While she plans to attend college, she is uncertain about the choice of a career, considering social work and biology. She is aware of emancipation conflicts with her parents: "I want to get out, yet I depend on them more than ever, yet I want to do things for myself and think on my own." She complains of nervousness before tests, mild anxiety in the dark, and occasional gastrointestinal upsets. She may be somewhat overconcerned about her health, going to see the doctor when she has these upsets. On examination, she relates well; there is no affect or thinking disorder; and abstractions, memory, and concentration are good. There is little evidence of anxiety and no evidence of depression.

Past History: Birth and early development were normal. She had a skin rash from birth to age four, and several episodes of stepping on cracks in the pavement as a child. She had poor appetite until age thirteen and frequent colds until age ten. She was a tomboy until early adolescence. Menarche occurred at age fourteen, without difficulty, the patient having received information about it from both mother and school.

Family History: The mother is forty-nine, a housewife, an intelligent, warm, outgoing person, proud of her children, her husband, and their life together. Ann describes her mother as "wonderful, marvelous," a person whom she can talk to easily. Father is fifty-one, a successful businessman, who is tense and irritable, has an ulcer, and tends to be somewhat rigid and restrictive. Ann feels that he is interested in her but that he is stubborn. She argues with him, preferring to bring her problems to her mother. The mother, having been raised strictly, has always given Ann a good deal of freedom, which at times has created conflicts with the father, whose attitude is more restrictive. She has a brother aged twenty-six, who is married and out of the home, and a brother aged nine, who lives at home, and with both she has a good relationship.

Symptomatology, functioning, demographic factors, and family relationship in the two groups are examined below.

Symptoms

Let us emphasize that the subjects were separated into healthy or ill on the basis of clinical judgment of all the material available on each case. Present symptoms were then compared on a descriptive level. Certainly in view of current theory we could have anticipated that the relatively healthy have considerable symptomatology without actually being psychiatrically ill. For example, an adolescent could have a psychoneurotic symptom without being psychoneurotic, or a schizophrenic symptom without being schizophrenic. Our scheme for coding symptomatology, described in the Appendix, was designed to pick up these symptoms, since it was descriptive and based on review of the presenting symptomatology only.

In Table 13, if we first compare the control (Col. 1) with the R.H. (relatively healthy) (Col. 2), we notice that the clinical selection of a relatively healthy group has eliminated four symptom patterns (schizophrenic, hypochondriacal, psychophysiologic, and immature), markedly reduced two (acting-out, sexual difficulty), and substantially reduced two others (anxiety, depression). The differences between the control (Col. 1) and the P.I. (psychiatrically ill) (Col. 3) have been

Table 13.   Symptom Patterns: Control, R.H., and P.I.

Symptom Pattern	Col. 1 Control (N=101) (%)	Col. 2 R.H. (N=41) (%)	Col. 3 P.I. (N=93) (%)
Schizophrenic	5.9	0	24
Conversion	0	0	10
Hypochondriacal	3.0	0	15
Hysterical personality disorder	0	0	11
Psychophysiologic	1.0	0	8
Immature	14.8	0	19
Organic	0	0	1
Acting-out	18.8	4.9	50
Sexual difficulty	10.9	4.9	31
Anxiety	64.3	39.0	74
Depression	40.6	12.2	37
Phobic	10.9	7.3	8
Compulsive personality disorder	8.9	4.9	3
Obsessive-compulsive	18.8	14.6	5

presented in Chapter 13. If we now compare the R.H. with the P.I., we see that the R.H. contains no cases with the first seven patterns (schizophrenic, conversion, hypochondriacal, hysterical personality disorder, psychophysiologic, immature, organic). The next symptom pattern, acting-out, referred to in more detail later, shows a large difference between the two groups. The R.H. had several adolescents with temper tantrums, one who wanted to run away from home, but none with general negativism, rebellious behavior at school, overt hostility to parents or siblings, sexual acting-out, or delinquency. The next symptom pattern, sexual difficulty, also shows a big difference. Though there were two in the R.H. with sexual preoccupations, there were many more, almost a third, of the P.I. with actual sexual difficulties including sexual acting-out. The next two symptom patterns, anxiety and depression, though they reveal smaller differences between the two groups, are still two to three times more common among the P.I. than among the R.H. Depression differed also in intensity, a datum not reflected in the table. In the R.H. it was a mild, episodic affect, often expressed as feelings of inadequacy, while in the P.I. it was more intense, was more persistent, and often involved suicidal preoccupation and/or attempt. Though the anxiety symptom pattern was quite common in the R.H., one of its characteristics, i.e., autonomic symptoms of anxiety such as dizziness, palpitations, urgency, frequency, was much less prevalent than in the P.I., (R.H. = 4 per cent, P.I. = 14 per cent). The next two symptom patterns, phobic and compulsive personality disorder, are equally common, whereas the last, obsessive-compulsive, is greater in the R.H. than in the P.I.

As explained before, the examination of the R.H. differed from that of the P.I. in that they were given a questionnaire covering the entire spectrum of symptomatology, which increased the number of patterns detected. Again, however, these symptom patterns differed in intensity; in the R.H. they were mild while in the P.I. they were severe.

Impairment of Functioning

Table 14 compares the impairment of functioning of the three groups, control, R.H., and P.I.

Table 14.   Impairment of Functioning

Degree of Impairment	School			Social		
	Control (N=101) (%)	R.H. (N=41) (%)	P.I. (N=93) (%)	Control (N=101) (%)	R.H. (N=41) (%)	P.I. (N=93) (%)
Minimal	52.5	73.2	31.2	66.3	78.0	45.2
Mild	27.7	17.1	26.9	14.9	9.8	18.3
Moderate	19.8	9.7	16.1	11.9	9.8	12.9
Severe	0	0	25.8	5.9	0	15.0
Nonclassified	0	0	0	0	2.4	7.5
Unknown	0	0	0	1.0	0	1.1
Average*	.67	.37	1.4	.57	.30	1.0

* The average was determined by weighting the impairments as follows: Minimal = 0, Mild = 1, Moderate = 2, Severe = 3, and getting an average for each group.

Observing first the average school impairment, we notice that the R.H. is one-half as impaired as the control and one-fourth as impaired as the P.I. In distribution, 10 per cent of the R.H. and 42 per cent of the P.I. show an impairment of moderate or more. Of the four in the R.H. who were moderately impaired, three were in early adolescence and were failing two midterms, with occasional records of failure in the past. The other was a sixteen-year-old high school junior, failing four subjects at midterm, with a past history of episodic failures in school though being promoted. The findings show that though school difficulty does occur in the R.H. it is more common and more severe in the P.I.

Turning to social impairment, and consulting the average first, we note that all three groups are less impaired in social than in school functioning, and again the social impairment of the R.H. is about one-half that of the control and one-quarter that of the P.I. In distribution, there are many more who are moderately and severely impaired in the P.I. (42 per cent) than in the R.H. (10 per cent). Of the four rated as moderately impaired in the R.H. group, two seventeen-year-old boys had recently moved (one to a new neighborhood, the other to a new college), so that they had few friends and no outside activities or close friends. The two others were young girls whose parents were quite restrictive about their social activities.

Demographic Factors and Family Relationships

Comparison of the groups for a number of factors revealed certain principal trends. Although the division of the two larger groups by health and illness could have altered the matching characteristics, they did remain the same with regard to age, sex, grade distribution, number of children in the family, and position of the adolescent in the family. The two groups, however, like the parent groups from which they came, differed somewhat in socioeconomic status (SES). Using income* as a guide, we found that approximately half of both groups came from the middle SES, but 40 per cent of the patients and only 10 per cent of the controls come from the lower SES, these figures being reversed for the upper SES. We attempted to control for SES by selecting the control adolescent from the same school as the patient.

---

* SES level was determined by income as follows: Low SES = less than $4,000 a year, Middle = $4,000–$7,999, Upper = over $8,000,

Many more subjects in the control group had fathers who were present in the home, and many more came from homes with both parents working, which may help explain the differences in SES.

When we studied family relationships, it became clear that these were two singularly different groups. The R.H. had grown up in a benign atmosphere. For the most part, both parents were present and, though they might have had considerable psychopathology themselves, they tended uniformly to have accepting and constructive attitudes toward their adolescents. Similarly, the adolescents were quite accepting of both parents and siblings. Conflicts, when they did arise, related to the adolescent's increasing need for emanicipation, i.e., more freedom with regard to dress, hours, dating, allowance. For the P.I. the converse held. Family relationships could be characterized as poor. There were fewer intact homes, with a higher proportion of absent fathers. Psychopathology of the parent often manifested itself in his relationship with the adolescent through domineering, rejecting, or oversolicitous attitudes. The adolescent was in marked and "chronic" conflict with the parent, the conflict relating to long-standing pathology on the part of both parent and adolescent rather than to current practical matters such as dress or dating. In addition, the adolescent patient was considerably more rejecting of his siblings.

Let us now discuss the impact of these findings. Although we had some difficulty, as indicated by the thirty-three controls classified as doubtful, when using traditional psychiatric criteria of illness, we were able to select clinically approximately half of a control group as relatively healthy. Though they may have had mild character disorder traits, or psychoneurotic symptoms, these latter tended to be single rather than multiple, of mild intensity, episodic rather than persistent, and not to impair their functioning. Diagnostically they ranged from symptom-free to mild psychoneuroses or personality disorders. These findings, suggesting somewhat more symptomatology than found by Offer [59, 60] in his study of normal adolescents, agree essentially with those of Grinker [34] and Golden [31] in that there was not an absence of psychopathology but little evidence of crippling or disabling illness. Though these relatively healthy adolescents may have sacrificed optimal dynamic integration for their adjustment, they functioned well scholastically and socially with many interests and activities, they came from intact homes, and they had positive relationships with parents and siblings. While considering this group healthy, we had several reservations as to whether they would also meet the psychoanalytic definition of normality described by Offer as utopian, i.e., harmonious blending of the diverse elements of the mental apparatus that leads to optimal functioning or self-actualization. Our information, based on one interview and without the aid of psychological testing, though adequate for a psychiatric definition of health, lacks sufficient depth to meet psychoanalytic criteria. In addition, many of the controls have just begun to deal with essential growth tasks of adolescence—emancipation and assumption of a heterosexual role—and may later develop more serious symptomatology when faced with resolving these tasks. Although their final status will have to remain in doubt until their developmental pattern has been completed, at this point they would have to be considered psychiatrically healthy.

When we compared the R.H. with the P.I., the differences were greater than those already shown between controls and patients. For example, the differences in acting-out are striking. Our finding of 5 per cent in the R.H. with acting-out is much less than Offer's (25 per cent with delinquent acts) and Grinker's (12 per cent with delinquent acts). In our group there were no delinquent acts. However, our findings do agree essentially with both Offer's and Grinker's final conclusions that there is very little rebellion in these adolescents.

These findings, together with those of Grinker [34], Offer [60], and Silber [71, 72], if supported by other work, suggest that serious modification of current theories, derived from the study of patients alone, of adolescent turmoil and its relationship to psychiatric illness, must be made. Again to use acting-out as an example, the marked differences between the two groups indicate that current theories about the significance of this symptom pattern in adolescence derived from the study of patients alone may have distorted its actual significance among healthy adolescents. Certainly in this latter group acting-out plays a minor role, and, to reiterate, without delinquent acts.

We do not, then, see a picture of adolescent turmoil simulating psychiatric illness.

SECTION VI

A SYNTHESIS

CHAPTER 15

THE PSYCHIATRIC SIGNIFICANCE
OF ADOLESCENT TURMOIL

> The wisdom of mankind creeps slowly on, Subject to every doubt that can retard Or fling it back upon an earlier time.
>
> —Richard Henry Hengist Horne:
> *Orion*, Book III, Canto II

TWO OF THE GREATEST INVESTIGATORS of this or any other century, Einstein [20] and Freud had a common conviction that science progresses, not only by patient, wormlike movements of investigation, but also by the soaring birdlike flights of theoretical speculation. In the foregoing fourteen chapters we have presented our own research steps together with careful reminders of the limits upon generalizations from our findings. In this chapter, cautioning the reader to remember that we are now dealing with theory rather than fact, we will free ourselves of the fetters of these limitations in order to (1) reevaluate the psychiatric significance of adolescent turmoil in the light of our observations, (2) present some clinical applications of our findings, and (3) indicate what questions remain unanswered and what are the most profitable and perhaps urgent directions for continuing work to take.

Let us briefly recapitulate current theory, which suggests that adolescent turmoil causes psychiatric syndromes to be vague, ill defined, and unstable and that often only later developments in the patient's life can disclose whether a given symptom picture represented pathology or merely the intensified difficulties of adolescence. Finally, it suggests that adolescent turmoil causes psychiatric symptoms to be common and transient in most adolescents.

How do our findings relate to this theory? We found that adolescent turmoil was at most an incidental factor subordinate to that of psychiatric illness in the onset, course, and outcome of the various conditions of our patients. Adolescence was but a way station in a long history of psychiatric illness which began in childhood and followed its own inexorable course, a course only temporarily colored by the developmental stage of adolescence. The decisive influence was psychiatric illness, not adolescent turmoil. The latter exerted its effect primarily by exacerbating and giving its own coloring to preexistent pathology. The decisive influence of psychiatric illness was clearly seen in the five-years-later study of outcome, when these patients had not grown out of their illnesses.

Our findings about diagnosis again run counter to theory. The difficulties in diagnosis lay, not in the choice between an adjustment reaction of adolescence and psychiatric illness, but in determining the exact diagnosis of the psychiatric illness. We could, however, support current theory at the initial interview when the sickness presented formidable diagnostic problems. But it soon became apparent that these problems were due more to manifestations of several clinical disorders in one clinical picture and unclear definition of the diagnostic categories than to anything related to adolescent turmoil. Without question, there is diagnostic difficulty which often is not resolved until time has passed, but it is not between turmoil and illness, and in truth does not seem to be related as much to turmoil as to some of the problems inherent in the manifestations of psychiatric illness. Furthermore, these patients, rather than showing unstable clinical pictures over the years, gradually tended to fit into more clearly differentiated and usual diagnostic categories.

Again, our findings seem to support the current theory in that symptoms are common among controls and patients. However, more careful scrutiny reveals that they actually qualify the theory; the symptoms among the controls tended primarily to be those of anxiety and depression and not the more serious psychiatric symptoms of schizophrenia and personality disorder.

Finally, the marked differences found between the relatively healthy and the psychiatrically ill adolescents, in symptomatology, functioning, and family relationships, point the way toward definition of normal progress through adolescent years—much needed by those who see large numbers of troubled young people.

What revisions of the current theory do these findings suggest? Although we must continue to view adolescent turmoil as a universal psychodynamic factor, its clinical psychiatric effects are surely far less significant than was previously thought. It plays a role subordinate to that of psychiatric illness in the sick and it is not so pronounced an influence as to blur the substantial differences between healthy and sick. Since its effects vary with different types of adolescents, they cannot be discussed in a universal or general sense. The psychiatric effects of adolescent turmoil may be viewed as a product of the interaction between the turmoil and the personality structure of the adolescent. In the healthy, whose personality structure is not only strong but flexible enough to withstand the onslaught, adolescent turmoil produces at most subclinical levels of anxiety and depression. In those with character neurosis, whose personality structures are rigidly organized with insufficient flexibility to respond to stress, it produces an acute clinical breakdown of psychoneurotic symptoms, which subside as the patient gets older, leaving a residue, however, of pathologic character traits. In those with schizophrenia and personality disorder, whose personality structures are loosely and poorly organized and who have the least flexibility to respond to stress, adolescent turmoil has its most chaotic effect by worsening the preexistent conditions, which then tend to persist into adulthood. In sum, then, the psychiatric effects of adolescent turmoil can be viewed as existing on a spectrum, with the healthy (on whom it has the least effect) on one end, those with character neurosis in the middle, and those with personality disorder and schizophrenia (on whom it has the most effect) on the other end.

How is this dramatic discrepancy between widely held theory and our findings to be explained? Have we set up a straw man? Our daily clinical experience with our patients and our exchange of observations with our colleagues tend to refute this supposition. In addition, the validity of the findings as well as our proposed hypotheses have recently been supported in an article by Alexander Gralnick [33], based on his clinical experience with adolescents over many years.

If we have not set up a straw man, how has this discrepancy come about? There are revealing clues in the original articles responsible for the theory [16, 19, 21–22, 24, 39]. We found that the authors shifted from describing a specific clinical problem in a patient to generalizing about adolescence as a stage of normal growth and development, without making quite plain to the reader that this step had taken place. Therefore, it is not always clear when the writer is talking about his findings in a patient and when he is propounding his theories about normal adolescence. It appears, then, that the theory of adolescent turmoil, derived presumably from the study of neurotics (although this is not spelled out either), has been inconsiderately generalized to all adolescents. This is obviously a crucial point since we found that the effect of adolescent turmoil varied so much, depending on the type of adolescent, that it cannot be generalized. The final pitfall is that the clinician, lacking psychiatric data to test the theory, and perhaps unaware of the extent to which findings on patients have been generalized to all adolescents, applies the generalization inappropriately and indiscriminately to his patients. Thus, since most of his patients probably suffer from either schizophrenia or personality disorder, the psychiatric significance of adolescent turmoil becomes overestimated. Clearly, the onus for this situation must be borne equally by both the psychoanalyst and the psychiatrist, the former for generalizing too widely from his patient population, and the latter for accepting these generalizations without developing adequate psychiatric data to test them.

We must now consider the work that remains to be done. A key question with regard to our study, referred to in the text several times, is whether we just happened to obtain a group who were unusually sick. Although we have attempted to answer this question as best we can and our impressions have been supported by several other clinicians, from the present study we can offer no figures to indicate the numerical aspects of the problem on the spectrum proposed above. This can really be done only by similar studies of other clinic populations. A more likely possibility, indicative also of another aspect of the work remaining to be done, is that our patients were actually sicker than those seen in other settings, such as prep school or college, where a psychiatrist is more readily available to consult for milder and more acute difficulties. These settings provide an ideal opportunity to further refine the concept of adolescent turmoil. We have studied adolescent turmoil primarily inferentially through the study of psychiatrically ill and healthy adolescents. There is great need for a study in just such a school setting, devoted to adolescent turmoil itself, its clinical manifestations, and its dynamic origins and to demonstrate or disprove its transient nature, in observations two to five years later. Our observed differences between healthy and sick adolescents in an urban setting require further corroboration from other settings. Furthermore, our observations must be held tentative until we have finished our follow-up study of the healthy adolescents, since many have just begun to deal with the essential growth tasks of adolescence and may later develop more serious symptomatology when attempting to resolve these tasks.

When we consider the clinical implications of this work, our thoughts turn to diagnosis. The findings themselves support the usefulness of the diagnostic scheme despite its limitations, since the differences among patients consistently followed diagnostic lines whether we studied family relationship, diagnostic difficulty, or outcome. The fact that the findings varied by diagnosis is also a strong argument for being quite clear about what kind of patient one is talking about and for not generalizing about all patients or all adolescents from one type. The diagnostic category for the majority of our patients was personality disorder and bears out the widely held belief that the majority of adolescent patients coming to see psychiatrists suffer from personality disorder. In view of the enormity of the diagnostic difficulties due to the clinical characteristics of personality disorders, one cannot help wondering how much adolescent turmoil has been bearing the burden for what belongs in the personality disorder category. In other words, the psychiatrist sees an adolescent with a personality disorder and lays the difficulties in diagnosis to the fact that he is an adolescent rather than that he has a personality disorder. The psychiatrist then permits himself to make his own misguided generalization about adolescent turmoil and the myth grows.

We now conclude our work by taking up some of the implications of the findings for the evaluation and treatment of the adolescent patient. Our patients were all clearly ill, had a poor outcome, and differed distinguishably from the relatively healthy. This fact warrants considering the possibility that, except in prep school and college settings where psychiatrists are more readily available, the referral of an adolescent to a psychiatrist may act as a selective factor removing him from the company of those in whom adolescent turmoil plays a significant role and placing him among those with psychiatric illness in whom adolescent turmoil plays only an incidental role. Therefore, in his clinical evaluation the psychiatrist should substantially lower his index of concern as to what part of the clinical picture is related to turmoil. The burden of proof should be on the psychiatrist to establish that it is not illness if it has that clinical picture and, finally, that such diagnostic categories as adjustment reaction of adolescence, often used as a refuge or wastebasket, should be used with great care and with far more precise definition.

The findings on psychotherapy—though they are impressionistic and though the results might have been quite different in the hands of a skillful and experienced therapist, as opposed to a resident—have some disturbing implications. According to current theory, analysis is contraindicated in an adolescent because of his unstable ego structure and treatment should be primarily supportive and directive with the goal of overcoming regression and putting the adolescent back on his growth track. However, our findings indicate that the growth process, if left to its own devices, does not iron out the adolescent's difficulties, does not place him back on his growth track.

Should we be satisfied with symptomatic improvement, with the attendant possibility of a later impaired adjustment? Or should we plan therapy as an intermittent procedure throughout a much longer period of time, over years perhaps? Or should we focus therapy on a more fundamental resolution of underlying conflicts and repair of ego defects? Is the latter even possible to undertake in an adolescent in view of his unstable and fluid ego structure? The clinician faced with patients who need help cannot await final answers to these questions. He must act. Therefore, I will conclude with a few thoughts on how this work has influenced our own clinical approach.

The therapeutic encounter is a crucial one for the adolescent. In this stage of development he suffers from a psychiatric illness which will plague him in some way the rest of his life unless there is a successful therapeutic intervention. I therefore consider that, unless I can prove otherwise, my patient has a psychiatric illness. I reserve the category of adjustment reaction of adolescence for very few patients— and for these only when I can specifically define it and assuredly eliminate other diagnostic categories. Furthermore, I assume that my patient will not grow out of his illness and that he requires treatment which should be both intensive, meaning two to three times a week rather than once a week, and specific, meaning the interpretation and working through of the presenting problem—be it separation anxiety or depression based on feelings of abandonment—in conjunction with the recognition and treatment of underlying defects in ego structure. The hazards of postponement of treatment, less intensive treatment, or too brief treatment far outweigh in my mind the costs in time and trouble of the course advocated here.

APPENDIX

A. SYSTEMATIC METHOD

Organization and Coding of Data

The material obtained from the initial interviews was organized into categories. Table 15 lists the variables for these comparisons, which are of two types: demographic factors, such as age and sex, and clinical factors, such as symptoms, family history, and past history. Through actual trial analysis of 101 cases, all the items were systematically defined and a coding system was developed. The reliability of coding schemes was tested by determining the percentages of agreement of two coders, who independently coded thirty-three cases. Most of the coding involved two categories of judgment: judgment of presence or absence of specific symptoms and judgment of presence or absence of the sixteen symptom pattern groups listed in Table 16. For these judgments, the range of agreement was from 48 to 100 per cent, with a median of 97 per cent. For four category judgments, such as school and social impairment (Table 15, 9a, b,), the percentage of agreement was 82 per cent. For a ten category judgment, such as duration of present illness (duration being divided into ten time periods) (Table 15, 4b), the range of agreement was 82 per cent, with a median of 86.5 per cent. For a sixteen-category judgment, such as the choice of principal symptom pattern, the percentage of agreement was 73 per cent. The material from the case record was placed on code sheets and then punched on IBM cards for analysis. As examples, age of onset has been described on pages 15–16, classification of symptomatology is given below, and school and social impairment are shown in Tables 18 and 19.

Classification of Symptomatology

The symptom classification attempted to codify all the symptoms found on examination as well as others selected from textbooks and

other sources. From this material, descriptive symptom pattern groupings were arranged. These clinically derived groupings resembled the
diagnostic categories of the American Psychiatric Association's *Diagnostic and Statistical Manual of Mental Disorders* [2]. They were
determined, however, by reviewing only the present symptomatology
without recourse to the rest of the history and were thus purely descriptive. Each symptom pattern contained several symptoms which
were considered characteristic of that pattern. If one of the characteristic symptoms of a particular grouping was recorded, the patient was
considered to have that symptom pattern.

Table 16 gives the symptom pattern groupings together with the
characteristic symptoms for two patterns, depression and acting-out.
After listing the symptom patterns, the psychiatrist used his clinical
judgment to choose the principal one. For example, a patient with
recorded symptom patterns of anxiety, depression, phobic, and acting-
out may have the last of these designated as the principal symptom
pattern. Where there was doubt as to which of two symptom patterns
was the principal one, we decided to give priority to the thinking disorder, next the anxiety pattern, and finally the depression pattern. If
this rule seemed to distort classification of the case, we coded the
principal symptom pattern as undesignated. In addition, to take into
account symptoms that either were found in more than one symptom

Table 15.   Categories for Analysis

---

1. Age
2. Sex
3. Classification of symptomatology
4. Onset of present illness
   a. Age
   b. Duration
5. Social adjustment
6. School adjustment
7. Family relationships
8. Symptom intensity
9. Impairment of functioning
   a. School impairment
   b. Social impairment
   c. Total impairment
10. Family history of emotional illness
11. Past history of emotional illness
12. Stresses
13. Treatment

---

pattern or were not characteristic of any symptom pattern, we organized a checklist of sixty-two miscellaneous symptoms, including such symptoms as concentration difficulty, obesity, and nightmares.

Table 16. Symptom Pattern Groupings

A. *Thinking disorder pattern*
This grouping will include the following symptoms:
1. Inappropriate affect (i.e., giggling, silly behavior, etc.)
2. Delusions (i.e., somatic, paranoid, etc.)
3. Hallucinations (i.e., auditory, visual, etc.)
4. Bizarre ideation
5. Bizarre motor behavior (i.e., inappropriate gestures, grimacing, etc.)
6. Mutism
7. Ideas of reference
8. Gross confusion of thinking
9. Disorganization of habits
10. Thinking disorder (i.e., looseness of association, concreteness, etc.)

B. *Anxiety pattern*
This grouping will include the following symptoms:
1. Anxiety (nervousness) up to panic reaction—generalized
2. Transient or intermittent autonomic symptoms, without organic etiology (i.e., dizzy spells, dyspnea, palpitations, nausea, diarrhea, polyuria)
3. Nail-biting, picking fingers; in general, repetitive motor behavior designed to relieve tension (including "restlessness")

C. *Conversion pattern and/or dissociation pattern*
This grouping will include symptoms of actual organic dysfunction where evidence of organic etiology is lacking. It will include the following symptoms:
1. "Anesthesia" symptoms (anosmia, blindness, deafness)
2. "Paralysis" symptoms (paresis, aphonia, monoplegia, hemiplegia)
3. "Dyskinesia" symptoms (tic, tremor, posturing)
4. Automatic behavior, fugue, amnesia
5. Other (conversion symptoms)

D. *Phobic pattern*
This grouping will include those patients suffering from a specific object or situational fear (i.e., fear of dirt, fear of closed places, fear of animals, fear of school, etc.).
1. Specific object or situational fear

E. *Obsessive-compulsive pattern*
This grouping will include the following:
1. Obsessive thoughts

E. *Obsessive-compulsive pattern* (Continued)
2. Repetitive, ritualistic acts (touching, counting, hand washing)
3. Compulsive speech
4. Other compulsions (i.e., compulsive eating)

F. *Depressive pattern*
This grouping will include patients with a pathologic affect of depression as manifested by the following symptoms:
1. Depression
2. Pathologic self-depreciation
3. Pathologic guilt
4. Suicidal preoccupation
5. Suicide attempt
6. Crying by history or crying during interview
7. Other (depressive pattern symptoms)

G. *Hypochondriacal pattern*
This grouping will include symptoms of somatic complaints and body overconcern without evidence of somatic dysfunction.
1. Somatic complaints without somatic dysfunction
2. Body overconcern

H. *Psychophysiologic pattern*
This will include symptoms of actual somatic dysfunction with organic pathology where psychogenic factors are considered predominant. The following conditions are among many possibilities:
1. Asthma
2. Migraine or tension headaches
3. Colitis
4. Other (psychophysiologic pattern symptoms, such as neurasthenia or fatigue states)

I. *Hysterical personality disorder pattern*
This grouping is characterized by "persons who are vain and egocentric, who display labile and excitable but shallow affectivity, whose dramatic attention seeking and histrionic behavior may go to the extremes of lying and even pseudologia phantastica, who are very conscious of sex, sexually provocative and who are dependently demanding in interpersonal situations." The following symptoms were included as characteristic:
1. Erotic or overdramatic behavior
2. Dramatic attention seeking
3. Overconsciousness of sex, sexual provocativeness
4. Histrionic behavior
5. Other (hysterical personality disorder pattern symptoms)

J. *Immature personality disorder pattern*
This grouping includes symptoms characterizing a late or delayed emergence from childhood, as follows:
1. Psychological immaturity (as manifested by childish speech, deportment, and activities)
2. Enuresis
3. Thumb-sucking

4. Trait of being easily picked on
5. Clinging to parent
6. Having friends younger than patient
7. Other (immature personality disorder pattern symptoms)
8. Excessive difficulty in separating from parents, making own decisions, and directing own life in an independent way

K. *Compulsive personality disorder pattern*
   This grouping is characterized by overconscientiousness and overinhibited behavior resulting in greatly restricted, pathologic work and play patterns.
   1. Overconscientiousness
   2. Overinhibited behavior resulting in greatly restricted pathologic work and play
   3. Other (compulsive personality disorder symptoms)
   4. General rigidity of attitudes
   5. Meticulousness
   6. Inability to make decisions due to excessive scrupulosity

L. *Acting-out pattern* (defined as behavioral expressions of conflict)
   1. Juvenile delinquency (destructive antisocial behavior)
   2. Stealing
   3. Temper outbursts
   4. General negativism
   5. Rebellious behavior at school
   6. Physical hostility to parents
   7. Physical hostility to siblings
   8. Overtly hostile behavior—other
   9. Antisocial behavior—other
   10. Pathologic lying
   11. Running away from home
   12. Window peeping
   13. Lack of impulse control
   14. Sexual acting-out
   15. History of arrests
   16. Alcoholism
   17. Drug addiction
   18. Rape
   19. Chronic friction at work with authorities or associates expressed in behavior
   20. Inadequate personality (chronic work and social difficulties characterized by inadequacy with respect to intellectual, emotional, social and physical demands; neither physically nor mentally grossly deficient on examination, but showing inadaptability, ineptness, poor judgment, lack of physical and emotional stamina, and social incompatibility)
   21. Sociopathic personality (antisocial)
       (Patients whose behavior is not such as to be coded as acting-out, but who are sociopathic, will be coded here. The category refers to the following manifestations: chronic social difficulties, narcissism, low frustration tolerance, manipulativeness, inability to learn from experience, seeking tension release by acting-out.)

M. *Sexual difficulty pattern*
   1. Masturbation
   2. Homosexual behavior
   3. Fetishism
   4. Voyeurism
   5. Sexual preoccupations
   6. Sexual deviation—other
   7. Other sexual acting-out (i.e., promiscuity)
   8. Other sexual difficulties (impotence, frigidity, specific inhibition of sexual impulses, masochistic or sadistic fantasies, excessive anxiety, avoidance of opposite sex)

N. *Organic reaction pattern*
   This grouping includes symptoms clearly and directly derived from organic brain disease.
   1. Psychiatric symptoms derived from brain disease

O. *Undesignated*

P. *Absence of symptom patterns*
   These symptom pattern groupings with their distinctive, special symptoms were augmented in most cases by one or more of a large group of other, more generalized symptoms (following):
   1. Tension
   2. Concentration difficulty
   3. Tremulousness
   4. Difficulty falling asleep
   5. Nightmares
   6. Obesity
   7. Immaturity (for age group)
   8. Poor hygiene
   9. Vain and egocentric attitude
   10. Labile affect
   11. Minor physical diseases (colds, headaches, etc.)
   12. Arrogance
   13. Irritability
   14. Demandingness in interpersonal situations
   15. Truancy
   16. Low intelligence
   17. Lying
   18. Grand mal epilepsy
   19. Petit mal epilepsy
   20. Poor judgment
   21. Anorexia
   22. Passivity
   23. Blunted affect
   24. Flattened affect
   25. Poor abstractions
   26. Vagueness
   27. Circumstantiality
   28. Blocking
   29. Poor comprehension

30. Loss of interest in school or work
31. Decreased school or work performance
32. Decreased social performance
33. Poor socialization (few friends)
34. Feelings of inferiority
35. Withdrawal
36. Overcompliance
37. Shyness
38. Loneliness
39. Conflict with or about mother or mother surrogate
40. Conflict with or about father or father surrogate
41. Unexpressed feelings of hostility
42. Accident-proneness
43. Apathetic attitude
44. Evasiveness, guardedness
45. Denial
46. Conflict with or about sibling(s) or sibling surrogate
47. Dating older men
48. Reading disability
49. Stuttering
50. Physical disease or defect (i.e., hemophilia)
51. Inarticulateness
52. Sterile history
53. Introversion or isolation
54. Confabulation
55. Conflict with or about peers
56. Suspiciousness
57. Perseveration
58. Religious conflicts
59. Poor school or work performance
60. Conflict with spouse (hostile and aggressive or passive and clinging)
61. Vagueness in goals
62. Convulsive seizures

*Table 17.   Symptom Intensity Rating for Depression**

Mild	Mild depressed affect on psychiatric examination; history of unhappiness and crying; pessimistic; guilty
Moderate	Definite, pervasive, depressed affect on psychiatric examination with or without crying; history of feelings of futility, self-depreciation, suicidal ideation or preoccupation, other depression
Severe	Markedly depressed, tearful, self-depreciatory, guilty; motor retardation on psychiatric examination; history of marked depression or suicidal attempt

* The percentage of agreement of two coders independently coding symptom intensity was 73 per cent.

Table 18.   School Impairment*

Minimal	Passing work
Mild	Barely passing, passing subjects on a reduced schedule, failing an occasional subject
Moderate	Multiple failures without being left back
Severe	Being left back, unable to attend school

* The percentage of agreement of two coders independently coding thirty-three cases was 82 per cent.

Table 19.   Social Impairment*

A patient was rated as having no social impairment if he had two or more friends, had some socialization with adolescents of the opposite sex, had at least one close friend, and engaged in activities outside the home that involved group participation.

Minimal	If he received a negative in only one of the above five areas
Mild	If he received two negatives
Moderate	If he received three negatives
Severe	If he received four or more negatives

* The percentage of agreement of two coders independently coding social impairment was 85 per cent.

APPENDIX

B. CLINICAL METHOD

The following forms were filled out, during the interviews, in order to arrive at uniformity of clinical observation. The first applies to the follow-up interview of the patient himself.

Doctor's Examination of Patient

Name:

Address:

Telephone:

School Year:

Work:

Age:

Marital Status:

Race:

Religion:

Date of Birth:

Place of Birth:

Name, Address, and Telephone of Nearest Relative:

Date of First Evaluation in Payne Whitney Clinic:

Date of First Follow-up Interview:

Today's Date:

Case #: _____

I. *Symptoms and Treatment*
   A. *Former presenting complaints:* "Can you tell me what your problems were when you first came here?"

B. *Interval history of past illness* (symptoms, intensity, frequency, duration; include pertinent negatives): "How have these been worked out—if they have?" Ask re each individual symptom.

C. *Treatment*: "Have you had any treatment with a psychiatrist or psychologist, or at a social agency or clinic of any kind?"
When:

Where (name):

D. *Current presenting problems*: "I am interested in knowing any and all problems you have now."

II. *Social Adjustment*: "I would like you to tell me something about your friends, and how you spend your time."

    A. *Number of friends*
        1. Many friends
        2. Few friends
        3. No friends
        4. Difficulty making friends
        5. Nonclassified

    B. *Sex of friends*
        1. Same sex
        2. Both sexes
        3. Nonclassified

    C. *Age of friends*
        1. Younger
        2. Older

      3. Both
      4. Peers
      5. Nonclassified

  D. *Intimacy of friends*
      1. Close friend or friends
      2. Frequent changes in "close friends"
      3. No close friends
      4. Nonclassified

  E. *Outside activities*
      1. No outside activities
      2. Present
      3. Nonclassified

  F. *Socialization with spouse*
      1. Outside activities together
      2. No outside activities together
      3. Nonapplicable

III. *School Adjustment:* "Can you tell me how you are currently getting on at school (i.e., grades, behavior, and relationship to peers and teachers)?"

  A. *Present school adjustment, academic functioning*
      1. Doing well
      2. Passing
      3. Marginal (not up to grade, reading problem, "special" and "ungraded" class, "reduced schedule," barely passing)
      4. Single failure
      5. Multiple failures
      6. Repeated grades
      7. Nonclassifiable

IV. *Work Adjustment:* "How have you been getting along in employment?"

A. *Status of employment*
   1. Unknown
   2. Employed
   3. Part-time employment
   4. Unemployed (for psychiatric reasons)
   5. Unemployed (for nonpsychiatric reasons)
   6. In military service
   7. Nonclassified

B. *Work functioning*
   1. Doing well in continuous full-time or part-time work
   2. Working intermittently for circumstantial rather than work difficulty reasons
   3. Steady full-time or part-time employment but with work difficulties
   4. Working intermittently for work difficulty reasons
   5. Changing jobs frequently for work difficulty reasons
   6. Unemployed most of the time for psychiatric reasons
   7. Unemployed continuously for psychiatric reasons
   8. Unemployed for nonpsychiatric reasons
   9. Nonclassified

V. *Family Relationships*
   A. *Attitudes of mother to patient*
      1. "How would you describe your mother's personality?" Probe.

      2. "How would you describe her attitude toward you?" Probe.

      3. "How do you get along with each other?" Probe.

4. "What does your mother think of your problems? Does she understand you?"

5. "How does your mother handle problems when they arise?"

6. "Is she interested in your schoolwork and/or job?" Probe.

7. "Is she interested in the things you're interested in?"

Check off the following re attitudes of mother to patient
1. Positive
2. Negative
    a. Active rejection (domineering, angry, nagging, restrictive, kinds of punishment—specify)
    b. Passive rejection (lack of interest)
    c. Overindulgent, oversolicitous, overprotective
    d. Unconsciously stimulating patient
    e. No insight into patient's needs
    f. Unable to set limits
    g. Trying to realize unfulfilled goals through patient
3. Ambivalent
4. Nonclassifiable

B. *Attitudes of patient to mother*
    1. "How would you describe your attitude toward your mother?" Probe.

2. "How do you feel about your mother?" Probe.

3. "What might she do to improve your relationship?" Probe.

Check off the following re attitudes of patient to mother
1. Accepting
2. Verbally accepting but rebellious in behavior
3. Ambivalent
4. Hostile—verbally
5. Hostile—physically
6. Overly compliant
7. Clinging
8. Passively rejecting (i.e., withdrawal)
9. Nonclassifiable

C. *Attitudes of father to patient*
   1. "How would you describe your father's personality?" Probe.

   2. "How would you describe his attitude toward you?" Probe.

   3. "How do you get along with each other?" Probe.

   4. "What does your father think of your problems? Does he understand you?"

5. "How does your father handle problems when they arise?"

6. "Is he interested in your schoolwork and/or job?" Probe.

7. "Is he interested in the things you're interested in?"

Check off the following re attitudes of father to patient
1. Positive
2. Negative
   a. Active rejection (domineering, angry, nagging, restrictive, kinds of punishment—specify)
   b. Passive rejection (lack of interest)
   c. Overindulgent, oversolicitous, overprotective
   d. Unconsciously stimulating patient
   e. No insight into patient's needs
   f. Unable to set limits
   g. Trying to realize unfulfilled goals through patient
3. Ambivalent
4. Nonclassifiable

D. *Attitudes of patient to father*
   1. "How would you describe your attitude toward your father?" Probe.

   2. "How do you feel about your father?" Probe.

3. "What might he do to improve your relationship?" Probe.

Check off the following re attitudes of patient to father
1. Accepting
2. Verbally accepting but rebellious in behavior
3. Ambivalent
4. Hostile—verbally
5. Hostile—physically
6. Overly compliant
7. Clinging
8. Passively rejecting (i.e., withdrawal)
9. Nonclassifiable

E. *Attitudes of patient to siblings*
   1. Siblings and age

     a.

     b.

     c.

   2. "How do you feel about your (sibling)?" Probe.

   3. "What might he (she) do to improve your relationship?" Probe.

Check off the following re attitudes of patient to siblings
1. Accepting
2. Verbally accepting but rebellious in behavior
3. Ambivalent
4. Hostile—verbally
5. Hostile—physically
6. Overly compliant

7. Clinging
8. Passively rejecting (i.e., withdrawal)
9. Overly competitive
10. Nonclassifiable

VI. *Interval Events*
   A. *Physical illness*
      1. Patient
      2. Parent
      3. Sibling
      4. Other
      5. None

   B. *Changes of family constellation*
      1. None
      2. Marriage of patient
      3. Marriage of parent or parent surrogate
      4. Separation, divorce, or desertion of parents or parents surrogate
      5. Death of immediate family member
      6. Patient leaving home for reasons other than marriage
      7. Chronic hospitalization for either physical or psychiatric reasons of immediate family member
      8. Birth of a child or children within the family constellation other than to patient or wife
      9. Birth of a child or children to patient
      10. Marriage and birth of a child or children to patient or wife
      11. Other
      12. Nonclassified or unknown

   C. *School*
      1. No change
      2. Entry into high school
      3. Entry into college
      4. Entry into commercial school
      5. Change of school other than entry into high school, college, or commercial school
      6. Quit high school
      7. Quit college
      8. Quit commercial school
      9. Nonclassified
      10. Other
      11. Unknown

D. *Sociosexual changes*
   1. None
   2. Bodily changes (includes appearance of secondary sexual characteristics)
   3. Menarche
   4. First sexual intercourse
   5. Love affair
   6. Homosexual activities
   7. Other
   8. Nonclassified
   9. Unknown

   (Note: Probe for sexual adjustment)

E. *Antisocial events*
   1. None
   2. Stealing without imprisonment
   3. Stealing with imprisonment
   4. Drug addiction
   5. Criminal assault (with imprisonment)
   6. Nonclassified
   7. Other
   8. Unknown

F. *Traumatic experience*
   1. Yes (specify)
   2. No

G. *Other*
   1. Absent
   2. Present (specify)

VII. *Dwelling Situation*
   1. Lives alone
   2. Lives with one parent
   3. Lives with both parents
   4. Lives with parent(s) surrogate
   5. Lives with spouse
   6. Lives with friend(s)
   7. Lives with spouse and patient's parent(s)
   8. Lives with spouse and spouse's parent(s)

9. In military service or at school
10. In hospital
11. Other
12. Unknown

VIII. *Children of Patient*
1. No children or pregnancies
2. One child
3. Two children
4. Three children
5. History of spontaneous abortion
6. History of illegal abortion
7. Children and pregnancy at time of interview
8. Children and history of spontaneous abortion
9. Children and history of illegal abortion
10. Nonclassified
11. Other
12. Unknown

IX. *Marriage and Children*
A. *Background (date of marriage, courtship)*

B. *Attitudes of patient toward spouse*
1. "How do you and your wife (husband) get along with each other?" Probe.

2. "How would you describe your wife (husband)? Do you think she (he) has any problems?"

3. "What does she (he) think of your problems? Does she (he) understand you?" Probe.

4. "Are the two of you interested in the same things?" Probe.

Check off the following re attitudes of patient to spouse
1. Accepting
2. Verbally accepting but negative in behavior
3. Ambivalent
4. Hostile—verbally
5. Hostile—Physically
6. Overly compliant
7. Clinging
8. Passively rejecting (i.e., withdrawal)
9. Nonclassifiable

C. *Attitudes of patient to children:* "Could you tell me something about your children?" (i.e., names and ages, behavior, relationships to you, personalities) Probe.

Check off the following re attitudes of patient to children
1. Positive
2. Negative
   a. Active rejection
   b. Passive rejection
   c. Overly indulgent, solicitous, protective, stimulating
3. Ambivalent
4. Nonclassified

X. *Psychiatric Examination*
   A. *Physical appearance*
      1. Size

      2. Grooming

      3. General impression (including degree of relatedness)

B. *Speech*
   1. Spontaneity (i.e., spontaneous, answers questions; pressured speech)

   2. Abnormalities of speech content

C. *Preoccupations* (including thinking disorder)

D. *Affect*
   1. Was the affect flat, blunted, or "normal"?
   2. Was the affect inappropriate (specify)?
   3. Depression
   4. Elation
   5. Anxious
   6. Tense
   7. Mood statement

E. *Abstractions*
   1. Idleness, laziness

   2. Misery, poverty

   3. Reputation, character

F. *Judgment* (plans): "What are your plans for the future?"

G. *Digit span*

Digits forward	Digits backward
582	629
6439	3279
42731	15286
619473	539418
5917428	8129365
58192647	94376258
275862584	

XI. *Examiner's Evaluation of Patient* (include statement as to present
level of adjustment with regard to functioning and the presence and
absence of symptoms)

Social Worker's Interview of Parent

This next form applies to the follow-up interviews with parents.

Name:

Address:

Telephone:

School Year:

Work:

Age:

Marital Status:

Race:

Religion:

Date of Birth:

Place of Birth:

Name, Address, and Telephone Number of Nearest Relative:

Date of First Evaluation in Payne Whitney Clinic:

Date of First Follow-up Interview:

Today's Date:

Case #: _____
Name: _____
Relationship: _____
Age: _____

I. *History: Interval and Current*
   A. *Interval history illness:* "Do you recall the problems your son (daughter) had when first seen here? Do you remember what

they were when we talked last? What do you think has happened to them? Are they still present? Better? Worse?"

B. *Current presenting complaints*: "Have any problems developed since then? How are they now? I am interested in all the problems, major or minor."

C. *Parent's current attitude toward illness and patient*: "How do you feel about his (her) problems? Do you think they are serious? How serious?"

D. *Treatment*
1. "Has your son (daughter) had any treatment with a psychiatrist or psychologist, or at a social agency or clinic of any kind?"

When:

Where (name):

2. "Has anyone else in the family, including yourself, had any treatment?"

Who:

When:

Where (name):

II. *Current Setting*: "Would you tell me something about your financial situation?"

A. *Family income*

B. *Family members who work, at what, earnings*

C. *Living quarters:* number of rooms

Where does the patient sleep?

"Has there been any change in your living situation within the past few years or a major change at any time? If so, specify."

D. *Dwelling situation (patient)*
  1. Lives alone
  2. Lives with one parent
  3. Lives with both parents
  4. Lives with parent(s) surrogate
  5. Lives with spouse
  6. Lives with friend(s) of same sex
  7. Lives with spouse and patient's parent(s)
  8. Lives with spouse and spouse's parent(s)
  9. In military service or at school
  10. In hospital
  11. Other
  12. Unknown

III. *Social Adjustment:* "Can you tell me something about your son's (daughter's) friends and how he (she) spends his (her) time when not in school (or at work)?" (Question for last known social adjustment if patient no longer lives at home.)

A. *Number of friends*
  1. Many friends
  2. Few friends
  3. No friends
  4. Difficulty making friends
  5. Nonclassified

B. *Sex of friends*
  1. Same sex

2. Both sexes
3. Nonclassified

C. *Age of friends*
   1. Younger
   2. Older
   3. Both
   4. Peers
   5. Nonclassified

D. *Intimacy of friends*
   1. Close friend or friends
   2. Frequent changes in "close friends"
   3. No close friends
   4. Nonclassified

E. *Outside activities*
   1. No outside activities
   2. Present
   3. Nonclassified

F. *Socialization with spouse*
   1. Outside activities together
   2. No outside activities together
   3. Nonapplicable

IV. *School Adjustment:* "How is your son (daughter) currently getting on at school (i.e., grades, behavior, and relationship to peers and teachers)?"

A. *Present school adjustment, academic functioning*
   1. Doing well
   2. Passing
   3. Marginal (not up to grade, reading problem, "special" and "ungraded" class, "reduced schedule," barely passing)
   4. Single failure
   5. Multiple failures
   6. Repeated grades
   7. Nonclassifiable

V. *Work Adjustment:* "How has your son (daughter) been getting along in employment?"

A. *Status of employment*
   1. Unknown
   2. Employed
   3. Part-time employment
   4. Unemployed (for psychiatric reasons)
   5. Unemployed (for nonpsychiatric reasons)
   6. In military service
   7. Nonclassified

B. *Work functioning*
   1. Doing well in continuous full-time or part-time work
   2. Working intermittently for circumstantial rather than work difficulty reasons
   3. Steady full-time or part-time employment but with work difficulties
   4. Working intermittently for work difficulty reasons
   5. Changing jobs frequently for work difficulty reasons
   6. Unemployed most of the time for psychiatric reasons
   7. Unemployed continuously for psychiatric reasons
   8. Unemployed for nonpsychiatric reasons
   9. Nonclassified

VI. *Family Relationships:* "Now I'd like to ask you some questions about your family. Could you tell me how they get along with each other?"

A. *Mother*
   1. "How would you describe your personality? What sort of person are you?"

2. "How do you handle problems that arise at home?"

3. "Are you critical?"

B. *Attitudes of mother to patient*
   1. "How would you describe your son's (daughter's) personality?"

   2. "How do you and your son (daughter) get along together?"

   3. "What do you think of your son's (daughter's) problems? Does he (she) feel you understand him (her)?"

   4. "How interested are you in his (her) schoolwork and/or job, and how do you show this?"

   5. "Do you have any common interests?" Probe.

Check off the following re attitudes of mother to patient
1. Positive
2. Negative
    a. Active rejection (domineering, angry, nagging, restrictive, demanding, kinds of punishment—specify)
    b. Passive rejection (lack of interest)
    c. Overindulgent, oversolicitous, overprotective
    d. Unconsciously stimulating patient
    e. No insight into patient's needs
    f. Unable to set limits
    g. Trying to realize unfulfilled goals through patient
3. Ambivalent
4. Nonclassifiable

C. *Attitude of patient to mother*
    1. "How do you think your son (daughter) feels about you?" Probe.

    2. "What do you think you might do to improve your relationship?" Probe.

    Check off the following re attitudes of patient to mother
    1. Accepting
    2. Verbally accepting but rebellious in behavior
    3. Ambivalent
    4. Hostile—verbally
    5. Hostile—physically
    6. Overly compliant
    7. Clinging
    8. Passively rejecting (i.e., withdrawal)
    9. Nonclassifiable

D. *Father*
    1. "How would you describe your husband? What is he like?"

2. "How does he handle problems that arise at home?"

3. "Is he critical?"

E. *Attitudes of father to patient*
 1. "How do your husband and son (daughter) get along to-
    gether?"

 2. "What does your husband think of your son's (daughter's)
    problems? Does he (she) feel he understands him (her)?"

 3. "How interested is he in his (her) school work and/or job,
    and how does he show this?"

 4. "Do they have any common interests?" Probe.

Check off the following re attitudes of father to patient
 1. Positive
 2. Negative
    a. Active rejection (domineering, angry, nagging, restrictive,
       demanding, kinds of punishment—specify)

        b. Passive rejection (lack of interest)
        c. Overindulgent, oversolicitous, overprotective
        d. Unconsciously stimulating patient
        e. No insight into patient's needs
        f. Unable to set limits
        g. Trying to realize unfulfilled goals through patient
     3. Ambivalent
     4. Nonclassifiable

F. *Attitudes of patient to father*
     1. "How do you think your son (daughter) feels about your husband?" Probe.

     2. "What do you think he might do to improve their relationship?" Probe.

     Check off the following re attitudes of patient to father
     1. Accepting
     2. Verbally accepting but rebellious in behavior
     3. Ambivalent
     4. Hostile—verbally
     5. Hostile—physically
     6. Overly compliant
     7. Clinging
     8. Passively rejecting (i.e., withdrawal)
     9. Nonclassifiable

G. *Attitudes of patient to siblings*
     1. Siblings and age

        a.

        b.

        c.

     2. "How does your son (daughter) feel about his (her) siblings?"

3. "What might he (she) do to improve their relationship?"

Check off the following re attitudes of patient to siblings
1. Accepting
2. Verbally accepting but rebellious in behavior
3. Ambivalent
4. Hostile—verbally
5. Hostile—physically
6. Overly compliant
7. Clinging
8. Passively rejecting (i.e., withdrawal)
9. Overly competitive
10. Nonclassifiable

VII. *Interval Events*

   A. *Physical illness*
      1. Patient
      2. Parent
      3. Sibling
      4. Other
      5. None

   B. *Changes of family constellation*
      1. None
      2. Marriage of patient
      3. Marriage of parent or parent surrogate
      4. Separation, divorce, or desertion of parents or parents surrogate
      5. Death of immediate family member
      6. Patient leaving home for reasons other than marriage
      7. Chronic hospitalization for either physical or psychiatric reasons of immediate family member
      8. Birth of a child or children within the family constellation other than to patient or wife
      9. Birth of a child or children to patient
      10. Marriage and birth of a child or children to patient or wife
      11. Other
      12. Nonclassified or unknown

C. *School*
   1. No change
   2. Entry into high school
   3. Entry into college
   4. Entry into commercial school
   5. Change of school other than entry (see above)
   6. Quit high school
   7. Quit college
   8. Quit commercial school
   9. Nonclassified
  10. Other
  11. Unknown

D. *Sociosexual changes*
   1. None
   2. Bodily changes (includes appearance of secondary sexual characteristics)
   3. Menarche
   4. First sexual intercourse
   5. Love affair
   6. Homosexual activities
   7. Other
   8. Nonclassified
   9. Unknown

E. *Antisocial events*
   1. None
   2. Stealing without imprisonment
   3. Stealing with imprisonment
   4. Drug addiction
   5. Criminal assault (with imprisonment)
   6. Nonclassified
   7. Other
   8. Unknown

F. *Traumatic experience*
   1. Yes (specify)
   2. No

G. *Other*
   1. Absent
   2. Present (specify)

VIII. *Children of Patient*
   1. No children or pregnancies

2. One child
3. Two children
4. Three children
5. History of spontaneous abortion
6. History of illegal abortion
7. Children and pregnancy at time of interview
8. Children and history of spontaneous abortion
9. Children and history of illegal abortion
10. Nonclassified
11. Other
12. Unknown

IX. *Marriage and Children*
  A. *Attitude of patient to spouse*
    1. "Can you tell me something about your son's (daughter's) marriage and how it seems to be working out?"

    2. "How would you describe your daughter-in-law (son-in-law)?"

    3. "How do the two of them get along with each other?"

    4. "What does she (he) think of your son's (daughter's) problems? Do you think she (he) understands them?"

    Check off the following re attitudes of patient to spouse
    1. Accepting
    2. Verbally accepting but negative in behavior
    3. Ambivalent

4. Hostile—verbally
5. Hostile—physically
6. Overly compliant
7. Clinging
8. Passively rejecting (i.e., withdrawal)
9. Nonclassifiable

B. *Attitudes of patient to children:* "Could you tell me something about your grandchildren (i.e., names and ages, behavior, personalities, relationship to your son [daughter], how he [she] handles them)?"

Check off the following re attitudes of patient to children
1. Positive
2. Negative
   a. Active rejection
   b. Passive rejection
   c. Overindulgent, oversolicitous, overprotective, overstimulating
3. Ambivalent
4. Nonclassifiable

X. *Patient's Plans for the Future:* "What are your son's (daughter's) plans for the future?"

XI. *Psychopathologic Observations of Parent*
1. Anxious

2. Tense

3. Depressed

4. Tearful

5. Preoccupied (specify)

6. Thinking disorder (specify)

7. Insight (specify)

8. Other

XII. *Examiner's Evaluation of Mother* (include statement as to present level of adjustment with regard to functioning and the presence and absence of symptoms)

Questionnaire for Patient and Parent

The following questionnaire, designed to cover the whole spectrum of psychopathology and applicable to both patient and parent, was used in follow-up interviews.

Name:

Address:

Telephone:

School Year:

Work:

Age:

Marital Status:

Race:

Religion:

Date of Birth:

Place of Birth:

Name, Address, and Telephone Number of Nearest Relative:

Date of First Evaluation in Payne Whitney Clinic:

Date of First Follow-up Interview:

Today's Date:

Case #: _____

QUESTIONNAIRE

1. Are you considered a nervous person?

2. Do you ever get nervous about anything unimportant?

3. Are you constantly keyed up and jittery?

4. Are you ever troubled by "cold sweats"? Would you say:
   a. Often
   b. Sometimes
   c. Never

5. Do you often feel restless?

6. Is it sometimes hard for you to concentrate?

7. Do you have any trouble getting to sleep or staying asleep? Would you say:
   a. Often
   b. Sometimes
   c. Never

8. Are you ever bothered by nightmares (dreams which frighten or upset you)? Would you say:
   a. Many times
   b. A few times
   c. Never
   About what?

9. Do you ever get tense or nervous about certain situations or things, such as closed places, classrooms, etc.?

10. Do you bite your nails often?

11. Are you ever bothered by difficulty breathing when tense?

12. Do you feel that you are bothered by all sorts (different kinds) of ailments in different parts of your body?
    a. Often

b. Sometimes
c. Never

13. Do you ever have diarrhea when you're nervous or upset?

14. Do you suffer from constipation? Under what circumstances?

15. How often are you bothered by having an upset stomach? Would you say you have an upset stomach:
a. Not very often
b. Pretty often
c. Nearly all the time

16. Are you worried much about your physical health? (specify)

17. Do you worry much about your physical appearance? (specify)

18. Are you ever troubled with headaches or pains in the head? Would you say:
a. Often
b. Sometimes
c. Never

19. Do you ever get spells of dizziness? Under what circumstances?

20. Have you ever had any fainting spells? Would you say:
a. Never
b. A few times
c. More than a few times
Under what circumstances?

21. Do you have asthma?

22. Do you have migraine?

23. Do you suffer from colitis?

24. Do you have any serious physical disease?

25. Do you ever suffer, even temporarily, from blindness or deafness or loss of smell?   Under what circumstances?

26. Do you ever suffer, even temporarily, from paralysis or loss of your voice? Under what circumstances?

27. Do you ever have muscle spasms?

28. Do you ever have thoughts that keep coming back in your mind? Are they frightening?

29. Do you ever find yourself doing things in a repetitive way—like stepping on every line on the pavement when walking or counting every car you pass or washing your hands frequently?

30. How many hours do you study each night?

31. Does it bother you very much if for some reason you can't study the usual amount of time?

    Are you bothered if you don't turn out the usual amount of work each day?

32. Do you ever find yourself needing to dominate a conversation or keep talking even though you may be repeating yourself?

33. Are you ever sad or depressed?

34. Do you ever cry?   Under what circumstances?

35. Does life seem hopeless?

36. Do you ever wish you were dead and away from it all?

37. Do you ever feel guilty about anything?

38. Have you ever tried to kill yourself?

39. Do you worry a lot?

40. Do you ever get funny ideas or unusual thoughts?   What?

41. Do you think that people sometimes laugh at you behind your back?

42. Do you trust people, generally?

43. Do you think people usually mean what they say?

44. Are you alone most of the time?

45. Do you ever have the feeling you've heard voices that weren't there or anything like that?

46. Do you ever feel that anybody is plotting against you?

47. Do you have frequent mood swings?

48. Do you feel your parents or spouse do enough for you? If not, what ought they to do?

49. Is bed-wetting a problem for you?

50. Are you overweight?

51. Do people sometimes pick on you?

52. Have you ever been in trouble with the police?

53. Have you ever stolen money or things?

54. Do you belong to a gang?

55. How often do you get into fights?

56. Do you often lie?

57. Are you very touchy or irritable?

58. Do you get into many arguments with your parents or spouse?

59. Do you fight with your brothers or sisters?

60. Have you played hookey very often, or do you stay home from work often?

61. Do you lose your temper easily?

62. Do you do a lot of things on impulse?

63. Have you ever gotten into trouble at school or at work?

64. Do you get angry often?

65. Do you often feel angry without showing it?

66. Do you ever feel angry toward your parents or spouse without showing it?

67. Have you ever had convulsions? When was the last convulsion?

68. Do you have any difficulty reading?

69. Have you ever stuttered?

70. Do you like school or work?

71. Do you ever feel that most other people are better or smarter than you?

72. Do you prefer to be by yourself most of the time?

73. Are you shy?

74. Are you lonely?

75. Do you spend a lot of time thinking about yourself?

76. Have you ever lost your memory, even temporarily? Under what circumstances?

77. Do you think much about sex?   (specify)

78. Do you have any sexual problems?   (specify)

79. Have you ever been bothered by your heart beating hard when upset? Would you say:
    a. Often
    b. Sometimes
    c. Never

80. How about such things as appetite? Would you say your appetite is:
    a. Poor
    b. Fair
    c. Good
    d. Too good

81. Do you feel in good spirits?
    a. Most of the time
    b. Sometimes
    c. Very few times

82. Have you ever taken narcotic drugs?

Examiner's Evaluation of Patient (include statement as to present level of adjustment with regard to functioning and the presence and absence of symptoms)

BIBLIOGRAPHY

1. Aichhorn, A. *Wayward Youth*. New York: Viking, 1935.
2. American Psychiatric Association. *Diagnostic and Statistical Manual of Mental Disorders*. Washington, D.C.: American Psychiatric Association, 1962.
3. Andry, R. S. *Delinquency and Parental Pathology*. London: Methuen, 1960.
4. Ausubel, D. P. *Theory and Problems of Adolescent Development*. New York: Grune & Stratton, 1954.
5. Baittle, B. Psychiatric aspects of the development of a street corner group: An exploratory study. *Amer. J. Orthopsychiat.* 31: 703–712, 1961.
6. Bardona, D. T., Mackeith, S. A., and Cameron, K. Symposium on the in-patient treatment of psychotic adolescents. *Brit. J. Med. Psychol.* 23: 107–118, 1950.
7. Beck, A. T. Reliability of psychiatric diagnoses: 1. A critique of systematic studies. *Amer. J. Psychiat.* 119: 210–216, 1962.
8. Beck, A. T., Ward, C. H., Mendelson, M., Mock, J. E., and Erbaugh, J. K. Reliability of psychiatric diagnoses: 2. A study of consistency of clinical judgments and ratings. *Amer. J. Psychiat.* 119: 351–357, 1962.
9. Beck, A. T., Ward, C. H., Mendelson, M., Mock, J. E., and Erbaugh, J. K. The psychiatric nomenclature. *Arch. Gen. Psychiat.* (Chicago) 7: 60–67, 1962.
10. Beckett, P. G. S., Pearson, C. E., and Rubin, E. A follow-up study comparing two approaches to the in-patient treatment of adolescent boys. *J. Nerv. Ment. Dis.* 134: 330–338, 1962.
11. Bender, L. The concept of pseudopsychopathic schizophrenia in adolescents. *Amer. J. Orthopsychiat.* 29: 491–512, 1959.
12. Bernfeld, S. Über eine typische Form der männlichen Pubertät. *Imago* 9: 1923.
13. Bernfeld, S. *Vom dichterischen Schaffen der Jugend*. Wien: Internationaler Psychanalytischer Verlag, 1924.
14. Bernfeld, S. Über die einfache männliche Pubertät. *Z. Psa. Pödagogik* 9: 1935.
15. Bernfeld, S. Types of adolescence. *Psa. Quart.* 7: 243–253, 1938.

16. Blos, P. *On Adolescence*. New York: Free Press, 1962.

17. Bridge, E. M. *Epilepsy and Convulsive Disorders in Children*, New York: McGraw-Hill, 1949.

18. Carter, A. B. The prognostic factors of adolescent psychoses. *J. Ment. Sci.* 88: 31–81, 1942.

19. Deutsch, H. *Psychology of Women*. New York: Grune & Stratton, 1944. Vol. I.

20. Einstein, A. *The World as I See It*. New York: Covici, Friede, 1934.

21. Eissler, K. R. Notes on problems of technique in the psychoanalytic treatment of adolescents: With some remarks on perversions. *The Psychoanalytic Study of the Child*. New York: International Universities Press, 1958. Vol. 13, pp. 223–254.

22. Erickson, E. H. The problem of ego identity. *J. Amer. Psychoanal. Ass.* 4: 56–121, 1956.

23. Freedman, A. M., and Bender, L. When the childhood schizophrenic grows up. *Amer. J. Orthopsychiat.* 27: 553–565, 1957.

24. Freud, A. *Psycho-Analytic Treatment of Children* (1927). London: Imago Publishing Co., 1946.

25. Freud, A. *The Ego and the Mechanisms of Defense*. New York: International Universities Press, 1946. Chaps. X and XI.

26. Freud, A. Adolescence. In *The Psychoanalytic Study of the Child*. New York: International Universities Press, 1958. Vol. 13, pp. 255–278.

27. Freud, A. Clinical studies in psychoanalysis: Research project of the Hamstead child therapy clinic. In *The Psychoanalytic Study of the Child*. New York: International Universities Press, 1959. Vol. 14, pp. 122–131.

28. Freud, S. *Three Essays on the Theory of Sexuality*. London: Hogarth, 1953. Standard Edition, Vol. VII.

29. Gerard, R. W., *et al.* Nosology of schizophrenia. *Amer. J. Psychiat.* 120: 16–29, 1963.

30. Glueck, S., and Glueck, E. *Juvenile Delinquents Grown Up*. New York: Commonwealth Fund, 1940.

31. Golden, J., Mandel, N., Glueck, B. C., Jr., and Feder, Z. A summary description of fifty "normal" white males. *Amer. J. Psychiat.* 119: 48–56, 1962.

32. Goolishian, H. A. A brief psychotherapy program for disturbed adolescents. *Amer. J. Orthopsychiat.* 32: 142–148, 1962.

33. Gralnick, A. Psychoanalysis and the treatment of adolescents in a private hospital. *Science and Psychoanalysis*. New York: Grune & Stratton, 1966. 102–108.

34. Grinker, R. R., Sr. "Mentally healthy" young males (homoclites). *Arch. Gen. Psychiat.* (Chicago) 6: 405–453, 1962.

35. Hamilton, D. M., McKinley, R. A., Moorhead, H. H., and Wall, J. H. Results of mental hospital treatment of troubled youth. *Amer. J. Psychiat.* 117: 811–816, 1961.

36. Henderson, D. K. Discussion on prognosis of psychoses in adolescence. *Brit. Med. J.* 2: 1090–1095, 1923.

37. Holmes, D. *The Adolescent in Psychotherapy*. Boston: Little, Brown, 1964.

38. Jones, E. Some problems of adolescence (1922). *Papers on Psycho-Analysis*, 5th ed. London: Baillière, Tindall & Cox, 1948.

39. Josselyn, I. The ego in adolescence. *Amer. J. Orthopsychiat.* 24: 223–237, 1954.

40. Kasanin, J., and Kaufman, M. R. A study of functional psychoses in childhood. *Amer. J. Psychiat.* 9: 307–384, 1929.

41. Leighton, D. C., Harding, J. S., Macklin, D. B., Hughes, C. C., and Leighton, A. H. Psychiatric findings of the Stirling County Study. *Amer. J. Psychiat.* 119: 1021–1026, 1963.

42. Lorand, S., and Schneer, H. I. (Eds.). *Adolescents: Psychoanalytic Approach to Problems and Therapy*. New York: Hoeber, 1961.

43. Lorr, M., Klett, C. J., and McNair, D. *Syndromes of Psychosis*. New York: Macmillan, 1963.

44. Lustman, S. Some issues in contemporary psychoanalytic research. *The Psychoanalytic Study of the Child*. New York: International Universities Press, 1963. Vol. 18, pp. 51–74.

45. Masterson, J. F., Jr. Prognosis in adolescent disorders—schizophrenia. *J. Nerv. Ment. Dis.* 124: 219–232, 1956.

46. Masterson, J. F., Jr. Prognosis in adolescent disorders. *Amer. J. Psychiat.* 114: 1097–1103, 1958.

47. Masterson, J. F., Jr. Delineation of psychiatric syndromes. *Compr. Psychiat.* 7: 166–174, 1966.

48. Masterson, J. F., Jr. The symptomatic adolescent five years later: He didn't grow out of it. Presented to the American Psychiatric Association, May, 1966.

49. Masterson, J. F., Jr., Corrigan, E. M., Kofkin, M. I., and Wallenstein, H. G. The symptomatic adolescent: Comparing patients

with controls. Presented to the American Orthopsychiatry Association, 1966.

50. Masterson, J. F., Jr., Tucker, K., and Berk, G.   Psychopathology in adolescence: IV. Clinical and dynamic characteristics. *Amer. J. Psychiat.* 120: 357–365, 1963.

51. Masterson, J. F., Jr., and Washburne, A.   The symptomatic adolescent: Psychiatric illness or adolescent turmoil. *Amer. J. Psychiat.* 122: 1240–1247, 1966.

52. Meissner, W. W.   Some anxiety indications in the adolescent boy. *J. Gen. Psychol.* 64: 251–257, 1961.

53. Merenda, P. F., and Rothney, J. W. M.   Evaluating the effects of counseling after eight years. *J. Counsel. Psychol.* 5: 163–168, 1958.

54. Michaels, J. J.   Character structure and character disorders. In Arieti, S. (Ed.), *American Handbook of Psychiatry*. New York: Basic Books, 1959. Vol. I, Chap. 19.

55. Miller, L. C.   Short term therapy with adolescents. *Amer. J. Orthopsychiat.* 29: 772–779, 1959.

56. Milman, D. H.   School phobia in older children and adolescents: Diagnostic implications and prognosis. *Pediatrics* 28: 462–471, 1961.

57. Nomenclature of psychiatric disorders and reactions. *Veterans Administration Technical Bulletin*, TB10A 78. Washington, D.C.: Government Printing Office, Oct. 1, 1947.

58. Nunberg, H.   Character and Neurosis. *Int. J. Psychoanal.* 37: pp. 36–45, 1956.

59. Offer, D., and Sabshin, M.   The psychiatrist and the normal adolescent. *Arch. Gen. Psychiat.* (Chicago) 9: 427–432, 1963.

60. Offer, D., Sabshin, M., and Marcus, D.   Clinical evaluation of normal adolescents. *Amer. J. Psychiat.* 121: 864–872, 1965.

61. O'Neal, P., and Robins, L. N.   The relation of childhood behavior problems to adult psychiatric status: A 30 year follow-up study of 150 subjects. *Amer. J. Psychiat.* 114:961–969, 1958.

62. O'Neal, P., and Robins, L. N.   Childhood patterns predictive of adult schizophrenia: A 30 year follow-up study. *Amer. J. Psychiat.* 115: 385–391, 1959.

63. O'Neal, P., and Robins, L. N.   The relation of childhood behavioral problems to adult psychiatric status: A 30 year follow-up study of 262 subjects. *Scientific Papers and Discussions, American Psychiatric Association, District Branches Publications* #1. Vol. 7: pp. 99–117.

64. Passamanick, B.   Editorial: On the neglect of diagnosis. *Amer. J. Orthopsychiat.* 33: 397–398, 1963.

65. Rinsley, D. B., and Hall, D. D.   Psychiatric hospital treatment of adolescents. *Arch. Gen. Psychiat.* (Chicago) 7: 287–294, 1962.

66. Robins, L. N., and O'Neal, P.   Clinical features of hysteria in children with a notable prognosis: A two-to-seven year follow-up study of 41 patients. *Nerv. Child* 10: 46–71, 1953.

67. Robins, L. N., and O'Neal, P.   Mortality, morbidity and crime: Problem children 30 years later. *Amer. Sociol. Rev.* 23: 162–171, 1958.

68. Roth, D., and Blatt, S. J.   Psychopathology of adolescence. *Arch. Gen. Psychiat.* (Chicago) 4: 289–298, 1961.

69. Sands, D. E.   The psychoses of adolescence. *J. Ment. Sci.* 102: 308–318, 1956.

70. Serrano, A. C., McDonald, E. C., Goolishian, H. A., MacGregor, R., and Ritchie, A.   Adolescent maladjustment and family dynamics. *Amer. J. Psychiat.* 118: 897–901, 1962.

71. Silber, E., Hamburg, D. A., Coelho, G. V., Murphey, E. B., Rosenberg, M., and Pearlin, L. I.   Adaptive behavior in competent adolescents. *Arch. Gen. Psychiat.* (Chicago) 5: 354–365, 1961.

72. Silber, E., Coelho, G. V., Murphey, E. B., Hamburg, D. A., Pearlin, L. I., and Rosenberg, M.   Competent adolescents coping with college decisions. *Arch. Gen. Psychiat.* (Chicago) 5: 517–527, 1961.

73. Spiegel, L. A.   A review of contributions to a psychoanalytic theory of adolescence. *The Psychoanalytic Study of the Child.* New York: International Universities Press, 1951. Vol. 6, pp. 375-393.

74. Srole, Leo, Langer, T. S., Michael, S. T., Opler, M. K., and Rennie, T. A. C.   *Mental Health in the Metropolis—The Midtown Manhattan Study.* New York: McGraw-Hill, 1962. Vol. I.

75. Toolan, J. M.   Changes in personality structure during adolescence. In Masserman, J. (Ed.), *Psychoanalysis and Human Values.* New York: Grune & Stratton, 1960.

76. Toolan, J. M.   Suicide and suicidal attempts in children and adolescents. *Amer. J. Psychiat.* 118: 719–724, 1962.

77. Warren, W.   Some relationships between the psychiatry of children and adults. *J. Ment. Sci.* 106: 815–826, 1960.

78. Warren, W.   A study of adolescent psychiatric in-patients and the outcome six or more years later: I. Clinical histories and hospital findings. *J. Child Psychol. Psychiat.* 6: 1–17, 1965.

79. Warren, W. A study of adolescent psychiatric in-patients and the outcome six or more years later: II. The follow-up study. *J. Child Psychol. Psychiat.* 6: 141–160, 1965.

80. Warren, W., and Cameron, K. Reactive psychosis in adolescence. *J. Ment. Sci.* 96: 448–457, 1950.

81. Weeks, H. A. *Youthful Offenders of Highlands: An Evaluation of the Short Term Treatment of Delinquent Boys.* Ann Arbor: University of Michigan Press, 1958.

82. Wertz, F. J. The fate of behavior disorders in adolescence. *Amer. J. Orthopsychiat.* 32: 423–433, 1962.

83. Wertz, F. J. Adolescent underachievers—evaluating psychodynamic and environmental stresses. *New York J. Med.* 63: 3524–3529, 1963.

INDEX

Acting-out
    and adolescent turmoil, 153
    in control group, 148-149, 153
    control group vs. patients, 139-
        141
    fluctuation over time in patients,
        112-115
    personality disorder and, 67, 112-
        113
    psychoneurosis and, 112-113
    relatively healthy vs. patients,
        149
    schizophrenia and, 112-113
    symptom pattern, 167
Adjustment reaction of adolescence
    criteria for, 5
    final view of, 161, 162
Adolescent turmoil, 137-144, 153,
        157-162
    acting-out and, 153
    in controls and patients, 143-144
    current theory of, 157
    defined, 27
    effect on character neurosis, 31-
        32, 159
    effect on illness, 27-33
    and epilepsy, 31, 105
    in personality disorder, 30-31,
        118, 159, 161
    and schizophrenia, 6, 29-30, 58,
        159
    significance overestimated, 129-
        130
Adolescence
    end of, effect on personality dis-
        order, 118
    as factor in diagnosing personal-
        ity disorder, 62
    lack of previous data on, 5-6
Affect, blunted, 117
Aggression, 22
    in character neurosis, 128
    in personality disorder, 127
    in schizophrenia, 127

American Psychiatric Association,
    Diagnostic and Statistical
    Manual of Mental Dis-
    orders, 3, 5, 17-21, 60, 119,
    164
Anxiety
    in control group, 148-150
    control group vs. patients, 139-
        141
    fluctuation over time in patients,
        115
    relatively healthy vs. patients,
        148-150
    symptom pattern, 165
Asthma. *See* Psychophysiologic
    symptoms

Beck, A. T., on classification of
    mental disorders, 17-18
Blos, Peter, on prediction studies, 8
Bridge, Edward M., *Epilepsy and*
    Convulsive Disorders in
    Children, 94-96

Cases, selection of, 12-13
Character neurosis
    and adolescent turmoil, 31-32,
        93, 159
    age of onset, 28
    clinical features, 87-88
    dependency in, 128
    diagnosing, 89-93
    differentiating from personality
        disorder, 85-86
    and functional impairment or
        outcome, 120, 124-125, 128-
        129
    and pathologic parent, 41-44
    results of psychotherapy, 132,
        134
Character traits, compulsive, 115-
    116

Father. *See* Parents

Freud, Anna, on nature of adolescence, 7

Functional impairment, 21-22, 120-130
  in control group, 150-151
  control group vs. patients, 142-143
  defined, 119
  in personality disorder, 133-134
  relatively healthy vs. patients, 150, 151
  scholastic, 170
  social, 170

Hypochondria
  in control group, 149
  control group vs. patients, 139-141
  fluctuation over time in patients, 116
  relatively healthy vs. patients, 149
  symptom pattern, 166

Hysterical personality disorder
  in control group, 149
  control group vs. patients, 139-141
  relatively healthy vs. patients, 149
  symptom pattern, 166

Immaturity
  in control group, 149
  control group vs. patients, 139-141
  relatively healthy vs. patients, 149
  symptom pattern, 166

Improvement of patients, 130-134

Inadequate personality, 79, 81-82
  symptom pattern, 167

Josselyn, Irene, on diagnosis of an adolescent, 8

Migraine. *See* Psychophysiologic symptoms

Mother. *See* Parents

Obesity, 117

Obsessive-compulsive symptom pattern, 165-166
  in control group, 149-150
  control group vs. patients, 139-141
  fluctuation over time in patients, 115
  relatively healthy vs. patients, 149-150

Organic reaction symptom pattern, 168
  in control group, 149
  control group vs. patients, 139-141
  relatively healthy vs. patients, 149

Parents. *See also* Family relationships
  attitude of, 16-17
  of relatively healthy, 152
  examination of, 185-198, 199-206
  father, pathologic, 36-44
  mother
    hindering diagnosis, 61-62
    pathologic attitude in, 34-44
  pathologic, 34-44
    effect on passive-aggressive, 40-41
    effect on personality disorder, 38-41, 75-77

Passive-aggressive subtype of personality disorder, 79-80
  and adolescent turmoil, 30-31
  and pathologic parent, 38-41
  and schizophrenia, 50, 54-55

Patients. *See* Clinical observation

Payne Whitney Clinic, 23

Personality disorder
  acting-out and, 112-113
  adolescent turmoil and, 30-31, 118, 159, 161
  age of onset, 28
  and blunted affect, 117
  character neurosis, differentiating from, 85-86
  and dependency, 127
  and depression, 73-74, 110-111
  diagnosing, 60-66